PRAISE

ask
Wh
matt

"*Ask What Matters?!* provides an extraordinary collection of personal practices and insights that will help any professional to reduce stress and enhance well-being. Paul and David have done a superb job in writing a book that synthesizes research from multiple disciplines in a way that matters most. This book has the potential to change the lives of many people."

—Dr. Nick van Dam, Global Chief Learning Officer for McKinsey & Company
professor at Nyenrode Business University and co-author of:
You! The Positive Force in Change.

"In a world where people often struggle with career/life choices, *Ask What Matters?!* provides readers an insightful and practical approach for cutting through complexity, making empowered decisions based on core values. In today's go-it-alone society, what differentiates *What Matters?!* from other approaches is its emphasis on people supporting one another to make their best choices. To that end, the book provides valuable tools and frameworks for having courageous "*What Matters?!*" conversations at work, with family, and in the community at large. *Ask What Matters?!* is a game-changing book for the new millennium."

—Mary Beaulieu, Assistant Dean and Director,
Office of Career Advancement, Harvard Kennedy School

"*What Matters?!* is both a provocative question and a practical response. Paul and David have brilliantly captured both—the power of personal inquiry and structures in layers to pursue the answers with curiosity and courage. The book comes to life with stories of those who have come face to face with the title question. In today's often mindless rush to move on, this is a mindful pause, a way to stop and ask; listen and choose."

—Phillip Sandahl, Co-author of *Co-Active Coaching* and Co-founder, Team Coaching International

"In this marvelous book, David Garten and Paul Sherman provide a framework and tools for life-improvement. They encourage readers in a nonjudgmental, safe way to ask: What values are most precious to me? And how can I place those ideals at the forefront of my busy life? What's more, the personal integrity and compassion of the authors shine through on every page. Readers who approach *Ask What Matters?!* with an open heart will learn a tremendous amount about their own unique spirit and how to transcend obstacles—often self-imposed—that have been placed along life's path. What a gift!"

—Rabbi Neal Gold, Director of Content and Programming, Association of Reform Zionists of America (ARZA)

"With our lives more stressful than ever, *Ask What Matters?!* provides a robust framework for our busy students to navigate and reset competing priorities. The toolkit targets the essence of what holds us back from being our best selves by providing clear, actionable practices and great real-world examples. I believe that integrating these ideas into our everyday lives will further not only academic and career progress, but more importantly, our overall sense of well-being."

—Stephanie Khurana, Faculty Dean, Cabot House,
Harvard University

"The concept of "work-life balance," while once useful, may have passed its prime. Nowadays, it's just "life." *Ask What Matters?!* is the perfect antidote for the shift we all need to recapture productivity and happiness—quite a rush. The five practices of the framework are clear, easy to understand, and most importantly, don't let you off the hook in terms of taking action. I can't think of any person, stage of life, industry or demographic where it doesn't apply—it's human."

—Lisa Kelly-Croswell, Senior Vice President & Chief Human Resources
Officer, Boston Medical Center

ask WHAT?! matters

A Practical Approach To Your Total Well-Being

10/14/16

For Harrison—

Always live What Matters?! and watch the magic unfold.

Enjoy!

PAUL SHERMAN AND DAVID GARTEN

For information about this title or to order other books and/or electronic media, contact:
What Matters?!
20 Kimberly Lane, Provincetown, MA 02657
www.askwhatmatters.com
info@askwhatmatters.com

ISBNs:
Print: 978-0-9977347-0-6
eBook: 978-0-9977347-1-3

Printed in the United States of America

Cover Design: Jennifer Smith-Little
Interior Design: 1106 Design

We dedicate this book in loving memory to our parents:
Patricia and Henry Garten, and Norma and Arthur Sherman.
For their love and support, and for teaching us what matters.

CONTENTS

INTRODUCTION
What Matters?!

What matters? Good question, right? Well, we like to think so. What matters to us right now is sharing with you just what we mean by *What Matters?!* We also want to explain why we think it's an important question for you to ask and how it will improve your life, and maybe even the world.

When we talk about *What Matters?!*, we are referring to a set of navigational tools called the *What Matters?!* framework. The framework will help you make choices—both the big life ones and the small daily ones—so you can thrive more and stress less. The framework will help you move beyond coping and live a life that holds meaning for you and brings you well-being.

Well-being is not something that happens randomly. Well-being comes from a crystal clear awareness of what matters to you so that you can make the best choices and take the proper actions to live a grounded, centered, and fully engaged life.

The *What Matters?!* approach is about both *what* you do—at home, at work, in relationships, in all areas of your life—and *how* you do it. It's the way in which you walk the path that becomes your life. As the saying goes, "The journey is the destination."

WHY *WHAT MATTERS?!* WHY NOW?

Why do you need a set of navigational tools in order to live by what matters to you? Isn't it intuitive? Consider the following . . .

For many of us, life in the twenty-first century is almost intolerably complex and demanding. Working, earning, parenting, dealing with health issues—even playing and enjoying time with friends—can feel like endless tasks with little fulfillment and way too much stress.

Add in concerns about the future of the planet, the economy, and humanity in general and we're totally overwhelmed. Powerlessness sets in. At best, we go on autopilot, putting our heads down and plowing as best we can through each day's demands. At worst, we feel desperate, depressed, anxious, and alone. (Sorry, we don't mean to bum you out. Fear not. You'll see we are optimists at heart!)

Even the seemingly mundane parts of life are no longer simple. A trip to the grocery store used to be mildly stressful, navigating the parking lot and coping with the sometimes long lines. In today's world, however, even the pressure of something as simple as food shopping has increased exponentially. We are inundated by choices, and there's data to prove it.

Jeff Davidson, author of *The Complete Idiot's Guide to Getting Things Done*, writes, "Your everyday supermarket now carries roughly 40,000 items—twice as many as a decade ago. There are so many products, so many brands and sub-species of those brands, that no consumer is safe from the bombardment of choice overload."[1] These days there are ten types of Liquid Tide, fourteen varieties of Cheerios, fifteen types of Thomas' English Muffins, and fifteen kinds of Crest toothpaste.[2] Attention, store manager, meltdown in Aisle 10!

Nowhere epitomizes the overwhelming nature of today's world more than the workplace. Businesses and other organizations face an unprecedented level of competition and complexity, which leads to "doing more with less." And this is only going to get worse. According to *Business Insider*, since the recession of 2008, 86 percent of executives say their company now expects more of their employees, and 59 percent of employees feel more pressure.[3]

We're also surrounded by technology, which is supposed to keep us connected and simplify our lives, but instead it drains us with its constant demand on our attention—cell phones, e-mails, social media. Add in the twenty-four-hour news cycle from around the world and we spend much of our time overwhelmed by information. Believe it or not, we've created more information in the past few years than in all of human history.[4]

Okay, just to be clear, this book is not a condemnation of business, technology, or the myriad consumer products available. We, your authors, have both benefited from successful careers in the corporate world. We love our smartphones and laptops and live streaming and 3,000 cable channels as much as anyone else.

Our goal is to demonstrate how the complex modern world is causing us to react, or in other words, be acted upon, rather than empowering us to live mindfully. The *What Matters?!* framework is about getting you back into the driver's seat by enabling you to make mindful choices.

FURTHERING THE CASE

In the early phase of the *What Matters?!* approach, we didn't use the term *mindful choices*. Instead, we talked about increasing the joy in life. The typical response we got was: "Joy? Joy isn't even on my radar. I'd be happy with just not being stressed out all the time." With our extensive coaching, consulting, and workshops, we thought we knew how much stress is in the world, but until we started digging deep into the research, we didn't realize how truly out of control it's gotten.

According to the Statistics Brain Research Institute, three out of four Americans regularly experience physical symptoms of stress. Nearly the same number experience stress-related psychological symptoms.[5] And it's not only Americans. The World Health Organization says that stress is the number one health epidemic of the twenty-first century.

This sad state of affairs is not just true for adults. Unfortunately the average high school student today experiences the same level of anxiety as the average psychiatric patient of the 1950s.[6] What's more, five times as many high school and college students are depressed and anxious today than during the Great Depression.[7]

And, for all of you employers out there, take notice. The American Institute of Stress says that stress-related illnesses cost $300 billion annually in health-care costs and missed work.[8]

No one is immune. It doesn't matter if you're a one percenter or if you earn minimum wage or even if you stay at home with the kids. The bottom line is clear: there is a new, toxic baseline for the amount and kind of stress people consider tolerable in their lives, and it significantly undermines the quality of life for millions of otherwise healthy people.

Many simply accept this new normal—perhaps because they believe that they don't have a choice—but that's not okay with us. Is it okay with you?

WHERE DOES STRESS COME FROM?

How did we get into this mess in the first place? Time for a quick (very quick) history of evolution and neurobiology.

Humans are hardwired to detect and avoid danger. For our cave-dwelling ancestors, danger came in the form of woolly mammoths and saber-toothed tigers, very real daily threats that demanded constant vigilance. Their senses had to be on alert all of the time for potential attack. To aid survival, their bodies produced the neurotransmitters adrenaline and cortisol, which create a "fight or flight" response to perceived threats.

In addition to this hyper-awareness, survival back in prehistoric days meant sticking with other people. Living in a group helped humans find food, stay warm, and fight off threats from wild animals or other tribes. Getting thrown out of the tribe for any reason was fatal. Belong or die!

Fast-forward to now. Most of us, in the developed world at least, no longer have to fight to live. Access to shelter and food is widespread. However, our brains are still wired to be vigilant. Consider the predators that stalk us in the twenty-first century: fears of job loss and poverty, of illness, of embarrassment and shame, to name just a few. Who among us hasn't at some point been afraid of becoming homeless and penniless? And the fact that some people *are* homeless—in a world with such abundance—only exacerbates our fear.

We know that getting laid off or divorced, or even going bankrupt, isn't the same as dying. And we know that if we don't have as nice a car or house as the neighbors or aren't wearing the same style of clothes as our friends, we won't be cast out to fend for ourselves in the wild. But try convincing your cave-dweller brain of that.

Our twenty-first century fears inject us with the same neurotransmitters that drove our ancestors to fight or flee. But because there's no longer the threat of being eaten, no fight or flight occurs. The adrenaline and cortisol produced by our hypersensitivity to modern-day circumstances build up and have nowhere to go. The result? These chemicals lead to internalized stress, which manifest as many ailments, both physiological and psychological.

WORKING IT

We invite you to pause here and ask yourself, Where are the saber-toothed tigers in your life? And in what ways are they damaging your well-being?

Ready to fight off those tigers? If so, you've come to the right place!

A SOLUTION TO COMPLEXITY AND OVERLOAD

Now that we have shown how modern living can undermine our physical and mental well-being, we want to offer you a compass to navigate this new normal: the *What Matters?!* Framework. At the very least we are confident that it will decrease the stress in your life. And, our highest hope is that it will provide you a greater sense of joy and fulfillment.

We like to describe the *What Matters?!* framework as a human technology for helping people thrive in complex times. It provides a foundation for conscious and intentional living amidst the over-stimulation of today's world.

Consider the very first operating system of a computer, whether it be Windows or Mac. These systems offered only the most basic programs. But with every subsequent update, their sophistication and capacity increased, and they could deal with more intricacies. A PC from the '80s could not have handled the demands of streaming movies, running Skype, or playing today's graphically realistic games. The operating systems of today do so effortlessly.

Similar to our increasing expectations of computers, human beings have set themselves a high bar in the twenty-first century. We're supposed to immediately process a continuous and over-whelming stream of information, sift through a staggering number of choices, and keep up with a dizzying pace.

The *What Matters?!* "operating system" gives you the awareness and skills to handle the influx without burning out. It allows you to step back and become the mindful observer and author of your life based on what truly matters to you, rather than getting swept up in reacting to the overstimulation of our modern world.

What Matters?! consists of five practices and five mindsets. The five practices are: Stop and Ask, Reach In, Reach Out, Plan, and Act. The five mindsets are: Curiosity, Kindness, Self-honesty, Humor, and Gratitude. Chapter 2 provides an overview of each practice and mindset. The other chapters do a deeper dive into each of these components. The figure on the following page visually depicts the framework.

The "human technology" of *What Matters?!* is based on Paul's twenty-five-plus years of worldwide experience coaching and con-sulting individuals and organizations from all walks of life; David's work with community organizations and private businesses; our

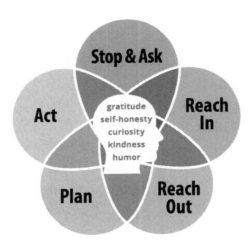

joint coaching of work teams; and our personal life experiences. The framework also incorporates many disciplines, including coaching theory, neuroscience, positive psychology, adult learning, twelve-step programs, Buddhism, Taoism, and leadership development.

What Matters?! has been successfully adopted by a wide variety of audiences—corporate executives, parents, young professionals, newlyweds, health-care workers, empty nesters, mid-lifers, retirees, and recent college graduates. The common denominator among these seemingly disparate groups is that they are all facing an unprecedented level of complexity. In short, the *What Matters?!* framework is universal. If you are a human being, you will benefit.

INSPIRATION FOR THE WHAT MATTERS?! APPROACH

The inspiration for *What Matters?!* stems from our own personal and professional life experiences, which we will share with you throughout the book. For now we'll focus on 2013, a pivotal year in our lives.

Days before the new year, Paul underwent emergency neck surgery. He had suffered multiple burnouts over his twenty-five-year career, and the stress had taken a physical toll. He was unable to work for some time after the surgery, so he spent his January and February laying on the couch in a hard collar. Nothing like the threat of paralysis to force you to stop and ask what matters.

Early in the year our close friend lost his father, Gerry, who was seventy-two. Although Paul was still recuperating and neither of us had met Gerry, we attended the memorial service to support our friend. What could have been a somber occasion turned out to be an amazing experience. To say Gerry was a character would be an understatement. We spent that February afternoon at the Falmouth Yacht Club, listening to Gerry's family and countless friends tell story after story of his infectious love of boats and the ocean. As we reflected on the drive back home, we agreed, "Boy, *that* was a life well lived!"

Later in the year one of our friends suffered a nervous break-down, provoked mostly by money worries. At around the same time, a second friend who had been unemployed for a year attempted suicide after being let go from his new job. Only a few years earlier, this same friend had beat stage 3 cancer. He had fought for his life then, but now he was willing to take it over a job.

On a September night when we reflected our friend's suicide attempt and the other's nervous breakdown, we sat on our sofa, dumbfounded. Was it just us or did it seem like the world was spinning off its axis? How could our friends have become so desperate? We could not grasp the juxtaposition of Gerry's long, well-lived life and the hopelessness of two young people.

Those incidents, coupled with Paul's health scare, were a wake-up call for us. With our new awareness, we realized there was a whole lot of *needless* suffering in the world—suffering that is internally generated or that is the inadvertent result of a choice. In other words, needless suffering is suffering that can be avoided: burnout, financial insecurity, fear of failure, keeping up with the Joneses, negative body image, road rage, performance pressure, bullying. The sheer amount of pain we saw was not okay with us and we wanted to put a stop to it.

Our friend and colleague Janelle Hoyland urged us to move forward with our goal. "Paul's struggles with burnout and your friends' hardships are emblematic of the world in general. New solutions for sustainability are required." Because of her encouragement, we created *What Matters?!* with the vision of ending needless suffering.

We realize that "suffering" is a strong word that may be hard for some to relate to, but stress is a rampant form of suffering. So, as you continue to read, we invite you to think about the stress in your own life and what is causing it.

WHAT THIS BOOK IS

Think of this book as an invitation. An invitation to explore a pragmatic and simple way to avoid distractions and stay focused on what is important to you. A guide to help you live a fully engaged life filled with well-being.

Throughout the book we will share our own stories as well as stories of our loved ones and our clients. These real-life examples illustrate the concepts of *What Matters?!* Some of the names have been changed for anonymity, but the stories are true.

We also have included sections called "Working It." These are opportunities for you to pause and reflect on the concepts. For those of you who like more in-depth, hands-on activities, we have provided a number of extended exercises to immerse yourself in the *What Matters?!* framework. Not into that sort of thing? Skip over them. They are by no means a requirement to benefit from this book. And you can always come back to them later; many are available on our website: www.askwhatmatters.com/resources.

Although we created the *What Matters?!* framework and some of the exercises, the book also contains a collection of other people's work. No need to reinvent the wheel when there is so much good work already out there. We consider ourselves to be curators in many ways, and we urge you to be one, too, as you choose the tools that work best for you.

It is our hope that you will become aware and stay aware of what truly matters to you. From this grounded place of awareness, we invite you to consciously choose how you live—daily, weekly, monthly, yearly. Since life is never perfect, you will still have to kiss some frogs along the way, but with mindful living, you will know how to correct your course, and you will be stronger for it.

WHAT THIS BOOK IS NOT

This book is not dogma. This book is not a panacea—we do not have all of the answers to the issues we are discussing. (By the way, did you notice that our framework is actually in the form of a question?) We believe that *you* are the best person to determine what type of life you want to live and how you want to live it.

We think of ourselves as a canary in a coal mine, signaling that this new normal of stress is deadly. We are simply a perfectly imperfect married couple who have had our own share of ups and downs, but we are truly blessed to have had far more ups. We have arrived here through a sometimes fearless and sometimes fearful examination of our own assumptions, expectations, and desires.

Our wish for you is to create a life filled with joy and absent of needless suffering.

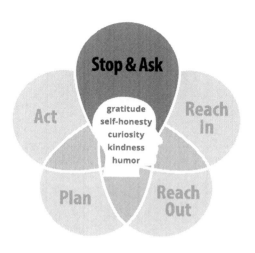

CHAPTER ONE
STOP AND ASK

In the January 2004 *Harvard Business Review*, Daniel Goleman wrote an article titled "What Makes a Leader," in which he highlights self-awareness as one component of emotional intelligence. According to Goleman, "Self-awareness means having a deep understanding of one's emotions, strengths, weaknesses, needs, and drives. Self-awareness extends to a person's understanding of his or her values and goals . . . someone who is highly self-aware knows where he is headed and why."[9] Self-awareness is the essence of Stop and Ask, the first of five practices we will present in the *What Matters?!* framework. We think there is no better way to achieve self-awareness than to simply Stop and Ask yourself the right question at the right time.

Stop and Ask is both the first of the *What Matters?!* practices and it is the foundation for the entire framework. When we take the time to Stop and Ask, we choose what to focus on, and just as importantly, what to ignore. Mindfully choosing will help you reduce stress and increase your well-being, creating a life that is sustainable.

Learning to make clear choices will help you live in alignment with what is important to you.

Stop

The process of living *What Matters?!* starts with stopping. That is to say, the first thing to do is slow down, whoa, hang on, halt, hold still, take a break, hit the pause button. Life these days moves a million miles an hour, and we just keep on trying to keep up. In fact, we make keeping up our highest aim: get the project done, get through the e-mail, get dinner on the table, get the kids up and dressed, get the deal closed, get through the workout, get going on vacation, get together with friends, get enough sleep. Even when we like what we're doing, we are nearly always under pressure to get something done, or worse yet, preoccupied with the next task. But with all that doing, we forget what it is we actually want—in other words, we forget why we got on this ride in the first place. The stress of the journey has erased the satisfaction of arriving at our destination.

"Stop and ask?" said Paul's friend Janet at their Harvard twenty-fifth college reunion. "I barely have time to stop and eat, stop and sleep, or stop and pee!"

You may feel like that, or you may be like our friend Nelson, who dismisses Stopping and Asking as woo-woo, New-Age navel gazing.

"Get real," Nelson says. "If we all spent our time contemplating this 'What's it all about, Alfie' crap, we'd have a lot of talk and nothing would get done."

However, a surprising set of evidence refutes the "I just don't have time" argument. Sociologist John Robinson, globally renowned for his extensive research on how people spend their time, said, "Time is a smokescreen. And it's a convenient excuse. Saying 'I don't have time,' is just another way of saying 'I'd rather do something else.'"[10]

If you're tempted to think, "Sure, easy for him to say," remember that he's not making this stuff up. He has half a century of research backing him.

Part of the negative attitude toward stopping comes from today's view of "busy." Being busy has become a status symbol and a defining component of self-worth. In fact, in our corporate coaching practice, we literally see people competing about being busy!

So at the risk of sounding redundant, what we're saying here is that the first step is to stop. Remember driver's ed? This is not a rolling stop, but a full stop. If all you have is five minutes, stop for five minutes. If all you have is two minutes, stop for two minutes. If you can spare a half hour, great! If you're always on planes, do it in the air. Stop making lists. Stop checking e-mail. Stop letting your mind wander. If possible, even stop thinking. Keep breathing, though.

There's a popular proverb that says, "In the end, your life will be immortalized on your tombstone with two dates, the date of your birth and the date of your death. In between the dates is a

Beware. If you can't find five minutes to stop, you might be facing what we call a What Matters?! Red Alert, a dangerous state where you are running so fast that either you've forgotten where you are going or you don't even realize that you've fallen prey to the frenzy of "getting there."

dash, and that dash is what matters."[11] Make the most of your dash. Make the time to Stop and Ask.

The Stop and Ask practice is actually fundamental to many different spiritual practices. Zen Master Thich Naht Hanh said, "We will be more successful in all our endeavors if we can let go of the habit of running all the time, and take little pauses to relax and recenter ourselves. And we'll also have a lot more joy in living."

If you can't identify with a Zen Master, consider the words of leadership authority Margaret Wheatly. "Without reflection, we go blindly on our way, creating more unintended consequences, and failing to achieve anything useful."

ASK

Now that you've stopped, it's time to ask. Ask yourself what really matters to you. What matters in this moment? What matters today? What matters this year? What matters in your relationship with your spouse? Your child? Your mom or brother? What matters in your community? What matters in that situation at work? Or in your upcoming conversation with your doctor?

You can then expand the reach of these questions. What matters to you in the bigger picture of your life? How are you spending your time? Is it working for you? What is going to make the difference for you between joy and suffering, satisfaction and disappointment, fulfillment and frustration?

What really matters? Ready to delve into this question? Try the following:

WORKING IT

Take a moment and reflect on your life and ask yourself, What matters to me? Seriously. Think about it. What really matters?

WHAT IF I DON'T KNOW WHAT MATTERS?!

What if you ask what matters but come up blank? You're not alone. Many of our workshop participants don't know the answer immediately. Fear and anxiety rear up, and that's okay. In fact, it's perfectly natural, as we humans have a deep "need to know." Uncertainty can cause discomfort, but not knowing an answer is different than not knowing the question.

Throughout this book you will find tools and exercises to help you first find the answers you have been seeking and then work with what you discover. Try them out and see what approach fits you best. Everything in this book is an invitation—an invitation to explore and choose what matters to you.

WHAT IF *EVERYTHING* MATTERS?

Once you've given yourself permission to Stop and Ask, it may seem that *everything* matters. If you find yourself unable to put one thing above another, here's a tip: focus your attention on something that is absolutely core to your own sustainable well-being. That's right. Put yourself first. If you think that's selfish and unworkable, here's another perspective: if the people in your life— your kids, your spouse, your best friend, your dog—depend on you for their well-being and you are not taking care of yourself in a way that is sustainable, you won't be able to reliably attend to their needs. As flight attendants say during their safety demonstration, "Put on your own oxygen mask first."

SOPHIE'S STORY: CARE FOR THE CAREGIVER

Sophie's husband, Calvin, was suffering from a third bout of cancer. Day after day Sophie dutifully accompanied Calvin to his treatments, sitting by his side for hours on end. She knew her presence comforted Calvin. In addition to caring for her spouse, Sophie was also facing the stresses of a teenage daughter and a demanding job.

Months of this routine began taking its toll on Sophie's physical and mental health. At her annual physical, Sophie's doctor warned her that she had to make some changes. She needed to allow herself time for the gym, for friends, and for other forms of self-care. Sophie realized that it was no longer sustainable to attend every one of her husband's treatments. Calvin was devastated; the way he saw it, she was choosing working out and socializing over him.

Though her initial guilt was excruciating, Sophie began replacing her visits to the hospital with other activities. Her physical and emotional health rebounded, and by taking care of herself, Sophie was able to navigate her life in a sustainable way. Honoring her role as wife and mother began with honoring herself. Thankfully, Calvin has since beat the cancer once again.

What Matters?! is about your own relationship with yourself. It's about what matters to you.

If you are grounded, centered, and taking care of yourself, you will be fully present in your life and able to attend to the people and things that matter to you. If, on the other hand, you are not taking care of yourself, no amount of time or money is going to allow you to engage in the other things that matter. We use the word *self-full* as a way of describing the effects of attending to our own well-being.

What Matters?! Is Personal

The question "What matters?" is deeply personal. There is no right or wrong answer. When you ask other people what matters to them, you may not like what you hear. But guess what? That's your problem, not theirs.

Paul's mother, Norma, had a wonderful saying that she lived by: "You don't owe anyone any explanations." She certainly walked that talk, proudly displaying her magna cum laude diploma from Radcliffe in the basement above her washer. That was her way of telling the world that motherhood was what mattered to her.

Nobody gets to tell someone else what should matter to them. Repeat *nobody*. You might not condone what matters to someone else, but as Pope Francis recently said so beautifully, "Who am I to judge?"

Want to be a billionaire hedge fund manager? As long as you do it legally, have at it. Quit your job and travel? Enjoy! Join an ashram and spend a year in silence? Good for you.

Okay, we know what you may be thinking. What if what matters to someone is bad or evil—to us or to most reasonable people? What about what mattered to Hitler or to bin Laden? What about what matters to terrorists? What about when discipline matters to a parent and it turns into abuse?

Let's clarify. In this book we are referring to personal choices that increase our own well-being—how we each spend our time and energy *in ways that improve our own lives.* When our choices encroach on other people without their consent, that's a different ball game. We've all signed up to be members of a civilized society. The cost of admission is adherence to basic laws and social norms. If you think those laws and norms are bad, put your energy into creating social change. Otherwise, consider your impact on those around you and choose responsibly.

Study after study has emphasized the strong human need to conform. Despite that instinctive urge, we implore you to listen to yourself and trust yourself. Ask what matters to you and act accordingly. In many cases, you may need to work with other people's needs or feelings as well as your own prior commitments. That's called being a responsible adult. It is, however, different than basing your decisions on other people's thoughts or opinions.

JANE AND ED'S STORY: AN UNCONVENTIONAL ENDING

Jane and Ed's marriage was a second for both of them, and each had grown children. They had been together for about twenty years and were ready to retire. They started the next act of their lives by spending half of the year in Cape Cod and the other half in Florida—a dream retirement for many. As time went on, Jane realized how much she loved Cape Cod and wanted to spend more of the year there, but Ed loved Florida and wanted to spend more time there. Both wanted to make the most of their remaining healthy, active years.

This was a Stop and Ask moment for them—where did they want to live? They had an honest conversation without blame or guilt. For Jane, Cape Cod was her true home, and she could see herself living there year-round. Ed felt the same way about Florida. In fact, they talked about how they were both starting to resent the time they were away from their preferred home.

What mattered to them in this phase of their lives was living in the place where they could thrive. So they decided to live separately for a year: Jane full-time in Cape Cod, and Ed in Florida. At the end of the year, they sat down and talked. Together they decided that they would both be happier living in their desired retirement location rather than with each other. They divorced—Jane took the house in Cape Cod and Ed took the condo in Florida. Some family and friends were a little bewildered by their decision, but Jane and Ed felt good about it, and still do.

What is your reaction to Jane and Ed's story? Confused? Sad? Disapproving? Our initial reaction was, "Wow, who would have thought of doing that?" Most people would have simply spent six months in their desired location and suffered through another six months in the other. What mattered to Jane and Ed, however, was being happy twelve months out of the year, and they were able to agree without either one suffering in the process.

This is a good time to talk about judgment. To start, let's differentiate judgment from observation. Observing is merely viewing whatever is going on, while judging is associating value or opinion to the situation. There are positive judgments like "that's one of the prettiest women in the room," and there are negative judgments like "what was she thinking wearing that dress?"

Science has proven that when we negatively judge others, we, the judgers, are actually causing ourselves physiological and psychological harm. A 2010 study in the Journal of Personality and Social Psychology warns that if you negatively judge others, you increase your risk for depression and various personality disorders.[12] (Not to mention the damage done to others.) Negative judgment is toxic. Do yourself and everyone else a favor, stop it! It will only take you off course from living what matters.

Let's consider an example of how judging someone can start. Say you get on a bus and a man weighing 400 pounds is taking up two seats and there is nowhere else to sit. You're exhausted from working all day and your compassion is at rock bottom. What might be going through your head? Maybe you start to envision what kind of diet got him to this weight (half a dozen donuts for breakfast, fast food for lunch, pizza for dinner, and two liters of Coca-Cola in between). Then you start to make up other things like (he's lazy, never exercises, and bet he tells everyone it's a thyroid issue). Then you start dictating silent prescriptions (go to the gym, eat a salad, and for pete's sake, walk to work occasionally), and you rationalize all of this by thinking "if you did those things, then you wouldn't be so fat and you would only need one seat, and you wouldn't be taking up my seat, too!" Whoa! Whoa! Alert! You just let yourself get mentally hijacked.

The reality is, you know nothing at all about this person. Yes, he is a certain weight and taking up two seats, but maybe he used to weigh 600 pounds. Regardless of what you think you know, when you negatively judge other people, you're actually causing yourself suffering. That guy on the bus is just sitting there contentedly, you are the one making yourself crazy with judgment.

Okay, we know what you might be thinking. Stop negative judgment? That's impossible! While it's certainly unrealistic to eliminate such a natural human tendency, later on we'll offer you some tools in the What Matters?! mindsets to help you resist the urge. In the meantime, suffice it to say that spending time negatively judging others prevents you from Stopping and Asking about yourself.

HONORING *WHAT MATTERS?!*

Once you take the time to Stop and Ask, you start realizing what matters to you. Now it's time to see how much *you* are honoring *What Matters?!*

Are you living in alignment with your principles? In other words, do your daily actions reflect what you say is important to you? If they are, that's great! We're going to help you continue to do so. If you aren't, don't beat yourself up. The remainder of this book is going to help you stay true to what matters to you.

You are constantly making choices in your life. Once you realize that every decision can be as easy as taking the time to Stop and Ask, then you see that the next choice is simply a matter of either living the life that matters to you, or not. Pretty simple concept, right? But it can be difficult to remember when you're constantly running and doing. That is why we call Stop and Ask a "practice." You need to practice bringing it into your daily life so it becomes a positive routine.

Accepting that you are always "in choice" can sometimes be difficult. There are simple choices, like choosing a glass of water over a soda or taking the stairs over the elevator, and there are harder choices, like choosing to leave a bad relationship or an unfulfilling job. But remember, in those last two cases, if you don't move on, you are still in choice—you are simply choosing to stay.

Now we invite you to look at the choices you are making in leading your own life. (Yes, we said "leading.")

THE *WHAT MATTERS?!* WHEEL™

Life is all about making choices. The purpose of the *What Matters?!* Wheel is to illuminate your own choices. This tool will show you whether the choices you're making are helping you live what matters to you, or not. So go ahead and take the *What Matters?!* Wheel™ for a spin.

The objective of this exercise is to give you a snapshot (or selfie!) of how you are doing living *What Matters?!* You will be asked a series of three questions and you will plot your answers on the diagram in Figure 2 on page 28. Once you've completed the diagram, you will see the areas where you are in alignment versus the areas that may need some work. The remaining practices in this book will help you discover the tools, resources, and people to help you live *What Matters?!*

Before you get started, take a look at the sample completed diagram in Figure 1. Don't worry about the numbers in the diagram. We just want to give you an example of what you will be doing.

Figure 1. Sample *What Matters?!* Wheel

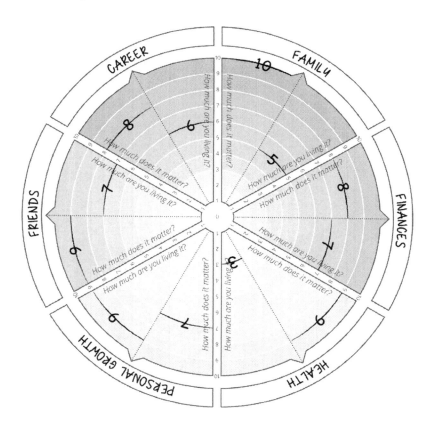

GETTING STARTED

Step One. First, Stop and Ask yourself what is most important to you, then jot down your answers in a list. This list will be an inventory of the most important parts of your life.

As you brainstorm, feel free to reflect on some suggestions for life areas in the table below. When you feel your list is long enough, select your top six areas—the ones that are most important to you—and write them on the outermost ring of each section of your wheel in Figure 2 on page 28.

LIFE AREAS			
Health	Self	Peace	Children
Family	Self-discovery	Volunteering	Clubs
Spirituality	Nature	Philanthropy	Fraternal organizations
Work	Music	Giving back	Career
Finance	Pets	Mentoring	Personal growth
Hobbies	Exercise	Sabbatical	Weight
Fun	Sports team	Leisure	Professional development
Friends	Work team	Joy	Athletics
Community	Charity	Love	Romance
Passion	Writing	Patriotism	Home buying
Art	Well-being	Neighbors	Mental health
Education	Politics	Entertainment	Fitness

LIFE AREAS			
Religion	Home	Relationships	Financial security
Retirement	Church	Sleep	Freedom
Parents	Religious groups	Creativity	Siblings

Step Two. As you consider placing each of your six components on the wheel, ask yourself, How important is each specific area to me? On a scale of zero to ten (zero being not important and ten being very important), pick a number that corresponds to each component's importance. Bear in mind, you aren't ranking these against each other, so you could have all tens or you could have all sixes, or any combination of numbers. On the left-hand side of the wedge for each area, mark the number that represents its importance.

Step Three. Look at the life components on your wheel and ask yourself, How much am I honoring this area of my life? Are the choices I'm making helping me to live this area of my life? Score each of the life components again on a scale of zero (not honoring) to ten (honoring completely) and write your response on the right-hand side of the corresponding wedge.

Looking at the wheel now, what do you see? What jumps out at you? Are you honoring the areas of your life that you say are important? Do your actions reflect your priorities? What are you feeling good about? What are you surprised about? Where do you need to focus your attention?

If you're feeling uneasy right now, you are not alone. Many of our workshop participants express a sense of guilt and negative self-judgment after completing this exercise. Try not to beat yourself up. Instead, use this as an opportunity to observe and be aware. Judgment shuts you down. Stop and Ask is all about opening yourself up to an honest exploration.

We encourage you to revisit your *What Matters?!* Wheel throughout this book as we discuss the remaining practices and tools that will help you live *What Matters?!*

Figure 2. *What Matters?!* Wheel

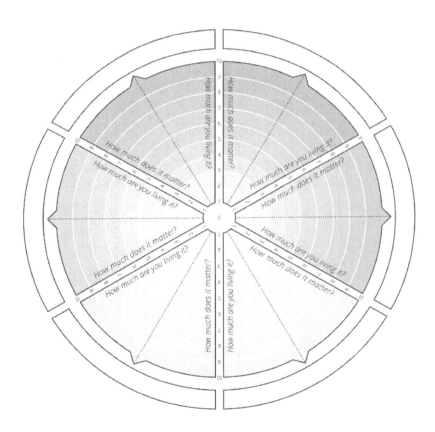

WHAT MATTERS?! LINGO

Before we leave Stop and Ask, we want to introduce some additional terms we'll be using throughout the book. They are designed to give you a shorthand as you work through the *What Matters?!* framework.

BIG AND LITTLE

We use the words *big* and *little* to differentiate the magnitude of what we are discussing. This terminology can be used throughout the *What Matters?!* framework, starting here with Stop and Ask. For instance, you might have a big Stop and Ask, like going on a retreat, or you might have a little one, like taking five minutes in the day to ask if you're living what matters to you.

STOP AND ASK MOMENT

During the Jane and Ed story, we said that they had a *Stop and Ask moment*. These are specific situations that require you to Stop and Ask what matters. A Stop and Ask moment can be caused by something as joyful as the birth of a child, or it can be brought on by misfortune, such as a job loss or an illness. Paul's neck surgery, for example, was a Stop and Ask moment, which eventually led to the writing of this book. Regardless of their origin, they require conscious and deliberate consideration of your priorities, choices, and behaviors.

WORKING IT

✓ Reflect on your life. Can you identify a Stop and Ask moment? What was the situation? How did it impact you? What role did it play in the choices you've made?

CHRISTINE'S STORY: CHOOSING THE TREADMILL

Christine is an executive at a large information technology company and she's responsible for a major division of the organization. Her job requires a lot of travel and inherently comes with a lot of stress. She had advanced many times in her five years on the job and felt financially secure, earning more than she had ever expected in her career.

Christine had recently been offered yet another promotion, which would involve longer hours and more travel. She came to us for a coaching session to help her walk through the possible repercussions.

When we asked her What Matters?!, *she responded without hesitation: "my family." She was happily married and had two great children. She also had a loving and supportive extended family and was blessed with many amazing friends.*

We asked her on a scale of zero to ten, with zero being "not much" and ten being "the most," to rate how important her family was compared to what else mattered to her. Her response was ten. Then we asked her how well she was honoring her family. We clarified by asking how she would rate her daily actions and choices as they reflected on her family being a ten. She furrowed her brow and said, "Well, if I'm being completely honest, I would have to say that even though my family is a ten, I am living it more like a four based on the time we spend together. I've missed far too many school plays and Little League games. I'm lucky if I get one sit-down dinner a week with my husband and the kids."

For homework, we invited her to have a Stop and Ask *moment, to reflect on the disparity between how important she said her family was and how much she was spending time with them.*

At our next session she reported back, "My husband and I discussed this at length. While I'm not thrilled to be missing out on day-to-day life with my family, it's very important to me that I provide for my family at a certain level. This includes sending my children to private school and ensuring that they graduate from college debt-free. So, although it involves some additional short-term sacrifice, I'm going to take the promotion."

We probed deeper to be sure that she was clear about both the positive and negative consequences of her choices. She was confident that she was mindfully choosing and doing what was right for her at this time.

Would you have done something different? Maybe, but that's not relevant. What is relevant is if you are living what matters to you. Her life is her business.

CHAPTER TWO
THE WHAT MATTERS?! PROCESS

The *What Matters?!* framework consists of five practices, beginning with Stop and Ask. These practices allow you to regularly self-reflect, have open and courageous conversations, explore previously invisible options, and dare to make meaningful, life-affirming changes. When you actually focus on *What Matters?!*, you realize how much time you spend thinking, doing, and worrying about what *doesn't* matter. By regularly engaging in the five practices of the *What Matters?!* framework, you can mindfully choose where to focus your time and resources, and where to jettison thoughts, behaviors, and yes, even people who weigh you down.

SIMPLE VERSUS EASY

The concept of simple versus easy may seem obvious. Deep down we all know most of these five practices, but given the demands and pace of everyday life, we oftentimes forget to consciously and intentionally choose. So, the concepts are simple, but incorporating them into your daily routine takes practice.

Our hope is, with enough practice, the model will become second nature to you and keep you on a path of well-being. Check it out for yourself.

To get started let's take a quick look at the following image:

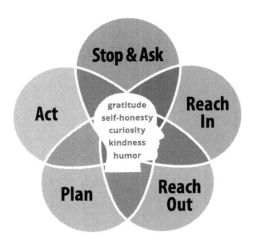

We will dig deeper into each practice eventually, but let's start with an overview. As you read through each practice, think about how you might consciously incorporate it into your daily, weekly, monthly, and yearly routines. Which practices come naturally to you? Which ones feel foreign? Our hope is that each one becomes a fundamental part of your life, like brushing your teeth or getting an annual physical.

At the end of each section will be a short quiz that will show how much you currently integrate the given practice into your life. Don't worry, you won't need a number 2 pencil, nor will you be graded. Your answers will simply highlight where you may want to pay special attention in later chapters.

It is important to point out that the *What Matters?!* framework is nonlinear. In other words, you don't have to do these practices in a particular order.

You can also find these questions online: www.askwhatmat ters.com/quiz.

STOP AND ASK

Don't let a day go by without asking who you are.

—DEEPAK CHOPRA, MD
FOUNDER OF THE CHOPRA CENTER FOR WELLBEING

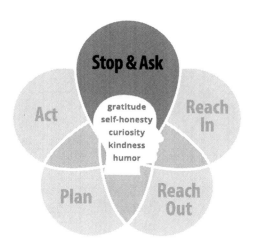

Since we've already talked extensively about Stop and Ask, we'll be brief here. Here you simply Stop and Ask yourself what's important: Am I living what really matters to me? Am I spending my time on what's important to me? Am I creating suffering or joy with my choices? And are these choices supporting or undermining my well-being? If you want to live *What Matters?!*, you need to pause—once a day, once an hour, as often as necessary—and ask yourself these key questions.

QUIZ

Read each of the following statements. Place a checkmark in the box that best describes your agreement with the statement.

I regularly stop and ask myself what is truly important.	Strongly Agree ☐	Agree ☐	Neutral ☐	Disagree ☐	Strongly Disagree ☐
I have a sense of purpose that guides what I do day-to-day.	Strongly Agree ☐	Agree ☐	Neutral ☐	Disagree ☐	Strongly Disagree ☐
Taking time for personal reflection is not optional; it is necessary for my well-being.	Strongly Agree ☐	Agree ☐	Neutral ☐	Disagree ☐	Strongly Disagree ☐

What was it like responding to these statements? What have you learned about yourself?

The more you answered "strongly agree" or "agree," the more you have developed your Stop and Ask capacity. The tools and resources in this book will help you deepen your practice. If you've found that these statements are not part of your repertoire, you'll have the opportunity to decide if and how you'd like to incorporate Stop and Ask into your life. The choice is yours.

Reach In

*We are disturbed not by what happens to us,
but by our thoughts about what happens.*

—Epictetus, ancient Greek philosopher

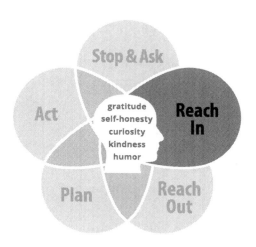

In order to live *What Matters?!*, you will need to Reach In and do whatever it takes to get in clear, grounded alignment with your body, mind, and spirit.

Note: We use the term *spirit* as that which is greater than our physical selves—you may choose the term *soul, heart, passion,* or whatever you are comfortable with. Remember, this is *your* process.

The goal of the *What Matters?!* framework is to increase your well-being. A key component of well-being is taking care of yourself. By Reaching In, you will learn how to build your resiliency. We talk about resiliency as a way of managing the people, thoughts, and things in your life that can cause you stress. Although you may not be able to change any of them directly, you *can* change how you relate and respond (not react) to them.

When we Reach In, we nourish our body, mind, and spirit, and we build our resiliency to overcome current and future circumstances. Reaching In can most simply be defined as: what you do to be comfortable in your own skin (and mind) so that you are in a healthy relationship with yourself and the world around you.

Examples of Reaching In can be as simple as eating a good meal, walking, dancing, journaling, listening to music, meditating, or praying. Whatever works for you, works! It's about calling forth your strength, being at your best, and getting centered so that you can get out of your own way and face any circumstance from a place of choice.

QUIZ

Read each of the following statements. Place a checkmark in the box that best describes your agreement with the statement.

	Strongly Agree	Agree	Neutral	Disagree	Strongly Disagree
I feel grounded in who I am and how I take care of myself.	☐	☐	☐	☐	☐
My negative self-talk rarely gets the better of me.	☐	☐	☐	☐	☐

I know what I need to do to recharge my batteries when I'm feeling depleted.	Strongly Agree ☐	Agree ☐	Neutral ☐	Disagree ☐	Strongly Disagree ☐
I accept, without frustration or resentment, that there are things in life that I cannot change.	Strongly Agree ☐	Agree ☐	Neutral ☐	Disagree ☐	Strongly Disagree ☐

What was it like to responding to these statements? What have you learned about yourself?

The more you answered "strongly agree" or "agree," the more you have developed your Reach In capacity. The tools and resources in this book will help you deepen your practice. If you've found that these statements are not part of your repertoire, you'll have the opportunity to decide if and how you'd like to incorporate Reach In into your life. The choice is yours.

REACH OUT

Alone we can do so little; together we can do so much.

—HELEN KELLER, AUTHOR AND POLITICAL ACTIVIST

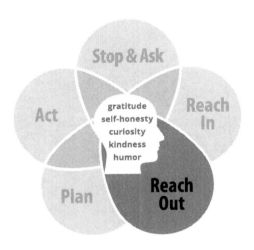

Reach Out is about finding the people who can help you live *What Matters?!* Who do you need beyond yourself in order to thrive?

Reaching Out can be very difficult for some of us. Unfortunately, as a society we have been taught to "go it alone." Asking for help is seen as a weakness, so we try to figure things out by ourselves. In reality, humans are like dogs: we are pack animals—it is in our DNA. Just ask our caveman ancestors. Without each other, they wouldn't have stood a chance in the tundra. A little too outdated an example for you? NFL quarterbacks have no problem asking their teammates for help blocking for them to give them time to make the right pass. Where would rock stars be without their backup singers and band? The irony is, when others ask us for help, we are not only happy to help, but we also feel a real sense of satisfaction in helping.

Reaching Out can be as simple as calling a friend when you are stressed. Or you can find a mentor, hire a coach, get a therapist, talk to your minister, priest, rabbi, imam/mullah, hairdresser, yogi, whomever! Join the club of your choice, whether it be a garden club, bike club, theater club, or book club. Whatever interests you—just get out there!

And don't wait for a crisis to Reach Out. Actively staying connected with others during nonstressful times builds a reserve of energy that you can mentally draw from when life gets difficult. Don't just take our word for it. In his 2014 book *Social: Why Our Brains Are Wired to Connect*, UCLA professor Matthew Lieberman cites research that shows having social connection is as important to health outcomes as not smoking.

A quick note: Although our book most likely falls into the genre of *self-help*, that's not one of our favorite terms. Not because we don't want people to help themselves (we do), but because we want people to also help each other. Though *self-help* is a well-meaning concept, it reinforces individualism and may unintentionally undermine interdependence, which allows us to thrive together as human beings.

That being the case, *What Matters?!* is a shared learning model designed to build community. We believe that we can all learn from, teach, and support one another. The Reach Out practice works both ways: it is meant for you to offer assistance to those in need as well as ask for help when you are in need.

QUIZ

Read each of the following statements. Place a checkmark in the box that best describes your agreement with the statement.

Although I have a group of family and friends, I often feel lonely.	Strongly Agree ☐	Agree ☐	Neutral ☐	Disagree ☐	Strongly Disagree ☐
It's easier to figure things out by myself rather than include others in the process.	Strongly Agree ☐	Agree ☐	Neutral ☐	Disagree ☐	Strongly Disagree ☐
When faced with challenges, I rarely turn to friends or family for ideas, advice, and encouragement.	Strongly Agree ☐	Agree ☐	Neutral ☐	Disagree ☐	Strongly Disagree ☐
I rarely call at least one friend or family member every day just to say hello.	Strongly Agree ☐	Agree ☐	Neutral ☐	Disagree ☐	Strongly Disagree ☐

What was it like to respond to these statements? What have you learned about yourself?

The more you answered "strongly disagree" or "disagree," the more you have developed your Reach Out capacity. The tools and resources in this book will help you deepen your practice. If you've found that these statements are not part of your repertoire, you'll have the opportunity to decide if and how you'd like to incorporate Reach Out into your life. The choice is yours.

PLAN

A goal without a plan is just a wish.

—ANTOINE DE SAINT-EXUPÉRY,
FRENCH PHILOSOPHER AND WRITER

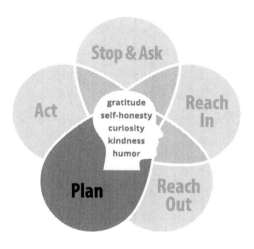

In our experience, living *What Matters?!* does not happen accidentally. It requires Planning. Every minute of every day we are choosing something, but we usually choose by default instead of with clear intention. It takes Planning to identify what you will do, when you will do it, and the support required to follow through. When you don't Plan, you end up reacting to the day's events as they occur rather than consciously and deliberately choosing where you want to go.

In a later chapter, we will delve into the practice of Plan as well as all of the other practices. Suffice it to say, if you want to reach your goals, you need to Plan.

Remember that small changes are a great way to start your journey. You don't have to boil the ocean. Also, the best plans focus on pursuing what is in your control while accepting (through the practice of Reach In) what is out of your control.

QUIZ

Read each statement below. Place a checkmark in the box that best describes your agreement with the statement.

I want to make changes in my life but am unsure how to proceed.	Strongly Agree ☐	Agree ☐	Neutral ☐	Disagree ☐	Strongly Disagree ☐
I seldom prioritize how I spend my time.	Strongly Agree ☐	Agree ☐	Neutral ☐	Disagree ☐	Strongly Disagree ☐
I'm often so busy it feels like my life is running me instead of me running my life.	Strongly Agree ☐	Agree ☐	Neutral ☐	Disagree ☐	Strongly Disagree ☐
I struggle with deciding what I will say "yes" to and what I will say "no" to.	Strongly Agree ☐	Agree ☐	Neutral ☐	Disagree ☐	Strongly Disagree ☐

What was it like to respond to these statements? What have you learned about yourself?

The more you answered "strongly disagree" or "disagree," the more you have developed your Plan capacity. The tools and resources in this book will help you deepen your practice. If you've found that these statements are not part of your repertoire, you'll have the opportunity to decide if and how you'd like to incorporate Plan into your life. The choice is yours.

Act

Don't sit in the waiting room of life.

—Dr. Seuss

By the time you get to the Act practice, you are ready to go and do what matters to you. Whatever you have decided, based on Stopping and Asking, Reaching In and Reaching Out, and Planning, *now* is the time do it. It is easy to talk yourself out of the steps you want (and need) to take in order to live what matters to you. Holding back while you wait for the perfect moment, the perfect words, or the perfect outfit will not work. Acting is about getting going and holding yourself accountable.

Remember the Nike slogan? "Just Do It!" We like to use that phrase when we explain the Act practice and the philosophy of imperfect action. It is better to Act on something that isn't quite perfect rather than never moving forward with any action. Once you are in action, you can always recalibrate as needed. As Albert Einstein said, "You never fail until you stop trying."

QUIZ

Read each of the following statements. Place a checkmark in the box that best describes your agreement with the statement.

I like to wait until everything is perfectly aligned rather than start and risk failure.	Strongly Agree ☐	Agree ☐	Neutral ☐	Disagree ☐	Strongly Disagree ☐
I seldom follow through on what I say I am going to do.	Strongly Agree ☐	Agree ☐	Neutral ☐	Disagree ☐	Strongly Disagree ☐
Most of my choices are based on what I fear rather than creating what I want	Strongly Agree ☐	Agree ☐	Neutral ☐	Disagree ☐	Strongly Disagree ☐

If I died tomorrow, I'd regret not having done what I really wanted to do.	Strongly Agree	Agree	Neutral	Disagree	Strongly Disagree
	☐	☐	☐	☐	☐

What was it like to respond to these statements? What have you learned about yourself?

The more you answered "strongly disagree" or "disagree," the more you have developed your Act capacity. The tools and resources in this book will help you deepen your practice. If you've found that these statements are not part of your repertoire, you'll have the opportunity to decide if and how you'd like to incorporate Act into your life. The choice is yours.

KATHRYN'S STORY: CHOOSING HEALTH AND LOVE

A few years ago Kathryn got a rude awakening about her life choices. She worked at home for a time-intensive client, becoming more stressed out, more isolated, and more overweight. She Stopped and Asked, "Am I thriving or simply surviving?" She did not like her answer.

Reaching In, Kathryn decided to start walking 10,000 steps a day. It meant getting out of the house and committing to her health. Soon, she started eating healthier foods. She also started a gratitude journal and set aside time each day to record what had gone well. She was feeling better and stronger.

Kathryn knew that her long-term partner, Chris, had always wanted to move to Cleveland. Kathryn loved California and had broken up with Chris a year prior, knowing that their relationship would be doomed when he decided to leave. One day she got a call from Chris. "Could you watch my cats while I house-hunt in Cleveland? My house sold in four days and I have to move quickly." Kathryn realized that if she did not reconnect with him, he would simply evaporate from her life without any chance for closure. She wanted more than that. So, she Reached Out to him and asked if she could help him pack his boxes.

In the short time it took Kathryn to help Chris, their relationship rekindled as if there had been no break. Chris asked Kathryn to marry him and move to Cleveland. She'd always pictured herself as a single, independent woman. California was home. Cleveland was cold and gray. She Reached Out to a few important friends in whom she could confide. The more she talked with them, the more she discovered that she wanted to move to Cleveland. She then made a Plan to follow her heart.

Kathryn's house sold in four days, and off she went to Cleveland with a shiny new ring on her finger. Even though the transition from California to Cleveland was bumpy, she found that Acting on her feelings helped carry her through.

Chris is a loving husband who supports Kathryn 110 percent. She lost fifty pounds and found lucrative employment that involves far less stress. Their home is a happy, relaxing place full of joyful surprises.

MINDSETS

The *What Matters?!* practices are intentional behavioral habits to enhance your well-being. To get their full benefit, however, there is an optimal state of mind to engage with yourself and the world around you. We call these the *What Matters?!* mindsets, If Stop and Ask, Reach In, Reach Out, Plan and Act are the engine of the

What Matters?! model, then the five mindsets: Humor, Kindness, Self-honesty, Curiosity, and Gratitude are the fuel (the rocket fuel) that propels you forward.

The *What Matters?!* mindsets offer another lens in which to view your world and any particular issue you may be facing. These mindsets are a consciously adopted set of attitudes, intents, and feelings that determine how we see and interpret the world around us. They are particularly helpful in changing your point of view when you are challenged by your circumstances. The field of positive psychology has proven that these mindsets open up possibilities and lessen negative emotions such as anxiety, jealousy, and aggression.

We invite you to incorporate the following five mindsets into your daily routine.

HUMOR

When did we all get so serious? Stop making everything so important and stop taking everything, including yourself and even *What Matters?!*, so damned seriously. Inject humor into your daily routine, and start by poking fun at yourself.

KINDNESS

It's sad that we even have to make an argument for kindness. For you cynics out there, research shows that kindness—both practicing it and receiving it—boosts your physical and mental well-being.

SELF-HONESTY

Tell yourself the unvarnished truth about who you are and what you want. Throw out of your lexicon *should* and *shouldn't* and *have to* and *can't*. Who are you trying to please, anyway? Be honest with yourself about things you've been avoiding in your life.

CURIOSITY

Look for what's beyond the obvious. Open your mind and explore the possibilities. Step outside of your comfort zone. Enjoy the childlike wonder that comes from suspending judgment. Who knows, you may just discover something new.

GRATITUDE

Gratitude is about expressing appreciation for what one has. Having a hard time feeling appreciative? How about starting by being grateful you can read this text?

One of the biggest benefits of adopting these mindsets is that you protect your mind from being hijacked and your body from hitting a minefield of adrenaline and cortisol. In short, these mindsets will reduce your stress, prevent needless suffering, and strengthen your resolve to stay true to what matters to you. An added bonus is that they will not only enhance your well-being but also the well-being of everyone around you.

SUE'S STORY: TURNING GRIEF INTO LEGACY

Sue is in a club that no one wants to be part of: parents who have lost a young child. Her son Kevin died of Sudden Cardiac Arrest (SCA) at the age of twenty while swimming at the lake with his friends on a beautiful July day. Initially thought to be an accidental drowning, the real cause of his death wasn't known until October when the coroner completed a full report. Sue and her family were devastated. Kevin was a star athlete, quiet, and always helped the underdog. He had opted to delay college because he wanted to hone his hockey skills in order to play for a

Division I or II school. Sue and her wife, Shannon, had supported Kevin and his decision.

Sue's grief was unbearable. She knew she had to keep going for her older son, Sean, who was in college at the time. She was also concerned about the potential strain it could have on her marriage. Shannon was the love of Sue's life and an amazing partner in every way, including raising their boys.

Sue tried to go on with her new life, but she noticed that even close friends didn't know how to be around her. Sue was at a crossroads: she could cling to her grief and become depressed or she could choose to do something to keep Kevin's memory alive.

This was her Stop and Ask moment. She resolved to do something positive to honor this amazing young man's life—but what could she do? When Sue read the coroner's report, she learned that Kevin's death was related to an undiagnosed condition: Hypertrophic Cardiomyopathy (HCM). HCM is a hardening of the heart muscle, which forces the heart to work harder to pump blood. In Kevin's case, his left ventricle was two-and-a-half times the size it should have been. Most people are never diagnosed, since screening is not part of a regular physical, and the symptoms, which include shortness of breath, dizziness, and chest pain, do not always occur.

Young athletes with HCM, like Kevin, are more likely to suffer sudden cardiac arrest because it can be triggered by intense physical activity. Sue Reached In and decided that helping to raise awareness about SCA could be her answer. What better way to keep Kevin's memory alive than to help other families avoid the pain she had to endure. This would be the ideal legacy to honor Kevin's kind and generous spirit.

Sue *Reached Out* to Parent Heart Watch, a national organization of parents whose children have died from or survived sudden cardiac arrest. There she found a place among families who understood how she felt. She learned more about the screening process that could detect those at risk of SCA, which typically strikes otherwise healthy young athletes like Kevin. She learned that the screening was not required to pass a high school physical for athletes. She also learned that in most cases of SCA, access to a defibrillator was the difference between life and death.

She put together a *Plan* that included raising awareness, promoting screening for HCM, and increasing the number and availability of defibrillators at youth sporting events. Sue *Acted* by starting the KEVS Foundation, which promotes awareness of the disease, offers free heart screening, and raises funds to buy defibrillators for sports teams.

Sue's goal is that every high school freshman in America will be screened for HCM. She also wants CPR certification and defibrillator training to be required for high school graduation. Her vision is that every time a team walks onto an athletic field, a defibrillator is as commonplace as water bottles.

CHAPTER THREE
WHAT GETS IN THE WAY

So far we have invited you to Stop and Ask and we have given an overview of the five practices and the five mindsets of the *What Matters?!* framework. Since the goal of *What Matters?!* is to decrease stress and increase well-being, we have intentionally created a process simple enough to work into your daily routine. Before we go any further into the individual practices, we first need to ask: What gets in the way of living *What Matters?!* This chapter will discuss some of those obstacles.

Basically, there are only two things that get in the way, and if you can learn how to deal with them, you are set to live a life filled with well-being. Are you ready? The two obstacles are: 1) you, and 2) EVERYTHING ELSE!

All kidding aside, it does come down to those two.

INTERNAL VERSUS EXTERNAL CIRCUMSTANCES

In the *What Matters?!* framework we define the "everything else" as your *external circumstances*. External circumstances are the things you have minimal or no control over, which may include the family you were born into, your native country, race, genetics, physical limitations, societal norms, and prejudices.

In addition, we can define external circumstances as those situations and responsibilities we have already stepped into, usually as a result of choices we made earlier in our lives, even as recently as last month! Perhaps you have a family to support, a business to run, or debts to pay off. Or perhaps you lack the education or experience to get the kind of job you would really like. Maybe you're married to someone who you now realize is not a good match for you. Maybe you travel so much for work that you no longer have any friends. Whether it is the boss from hell or the black mold in your attic, external circumstances are what many term "their reality": situations from which there is no turning back.

Often times we believe that our choices are limited because of our external circumstances—and yes, that can certainly be the case—but maybe we're also overestimating the power of our external circumstances. In other words, what if our barriers to well-being are, in fact, a function of our *internal circumstances*, the things we believe.

Internal circumstances are our thoughts and feelings. They decide how we respond to the world around us. Legendary singer Lena Horne said, "It's not the load that breaks you down, it's the way you carry it." The load she is referring to is external circumstances. But how you carry that load depends on your internal circumstances.

We will shortly delve deeper into what we mean by internal circumstances. Before doing so, we are compelled to share the following incredible story of a woman who navigated the most dire of external circumstances.

Catherine's Story: Choosing to Live While Dying

Catherine Royce, a former dancer, loving wife, dedicated mother of two, and our dear friend was diagnosed at age fifty-five with Amyotrophic Lateral Sclerosis (ALS), also called Lou Gehrig's disease, a lethal neurodegenerative disease that slowly paralyzes the body. Two-and-a-half years before her death, Catherine wrote an essay for NPR's "This I Believe" series.[13] In her essay she shares:

"I believe that I always have a choice. No matter what I'm doing. No matter what is happening to me. I always have a choice.

I have spent my life typing on a keyboard, but now I can no longer use my hands. Every day I sit at my computer speaking words into a microphone instead of typing. In 2003, I was diagnosed with ALS, Lou Gehrig's Disease. Over time, this disease will weaken and finally destroy every significant muscle in my body. Ultimately, I will be unable to move, to speak and, finally, to breathe. Already, I am largely dependent upon others. So every day I review my choices.

Living with ALS seems a bit like going into the witness protection program. Everything I have ever known about myself—how I look, how I act, how I interact with the world—is rapidly and radically changing. And yet, with each change, I still have choice.

When I could no longer type with my hands, I knew I could give up writing entirely or I could go through the arduous process of learning to use voice recognition software. I'm not a young woman. This took real work. Interestingly, I write more now than ever.

Every day I choose not only how I will live, but if I will live. I have no particular religious mandate that forbids contemplating a shorter life, an action that would deny this disease its ultimate expression. But this is where my belief in choice truly finds its power. I can choose to see ALS as nothing more than a death sentence, or I can choose to see it as an invitation—an opportunity to learn who I truly am."

Using her transcription software, Catherine spent her remaining time on earth chronicling her journey in a series of essays, which have been compiled into a book titled Wherever I Am, I'm Fine: Letters about Living While Dying. *You can find it on Amazon.*

As Catherine so bravely demonstrated, the more we actively shape our internal circumstances—our thoughts and feelings—the more we can make clear, empowered choices about our external circumstances. Learning to make those empowered choices is a core element of the *What Matters?!* framework. All this is to say, while we are certainly influenced by our external circumstances, we do not need to be held hostage by them. But try telling your mind that.

Laura Whitworth, a founder of the coaching profession, was one of Paul's mentors, and it was she who first warned him, "Your mind is like a dangerous neighborhood; don't go there alone." It's easy to succumb to misery and be walled in by negative thoughts and beliefs. In fact, it's estimated that 70–80 percent of our 60,000 daily thoughts are negative ones.[14] Even in their mildest forms, these negative thoughts feed the internal circumstances that prevent us from living *What Matters?!*

Take a look at the following list and consider how many of these negative recurring thoughts your mind might specialize in. Don't see some of your favorites on the list? Add them!

NEGATIVE THOUGHTS

- ☐ I'm lazy.
- ☐ I'll go broke.
- ☐ Why bother? Nothing is going to change.
- ☐ Who am I to (fill in blank)?
- ☐ No one cares.
- ☐ They'll laugh at me.
- ☐ I'm not smart enough.
- ☐ It's too risky.
- ☐ There's not enough time.
- ☐ I'm not working hard enough.
- ☐ Fast is good. Slow is bad.
- ☐ I'm irresponsible.
- ☐ They are better than me.
- ☐ I'm too fat.
- ☐ I don't have enough experience.
- ☐ I don't have enough money.
- ☐ It's too late for me.
- ☐ I don't know what I want.
- ☐ If I speak my mind, I'll be rejected.
- ☐ I should be further along than I am.
- ☐ I need to do more.
- ☐ If they really loved me, they would (fill in blank).
- ☐ Suck it up.
- ☐ I'm not doing it right.
- ☐ I'll never change.
- ☐ I need to please others.
- ☐ Failure is not an option.
- ☐ I don't deserve it (e.g., success, money, love).
- ☐ If only I had (fill in blank).
- ☐ It's just not fair.
- ☐ I'm too busy.
- ☐ I need fear to motivate me and keep me in check.
- ☐ I'm selfish.

INNER CRITIC AND NEGATIVE THINKING

These thoughts constitute our inner critic (or critics). Where do these inner critics come from? One explanation is that these critical voices come from ideas that were designed to protect you early in your life but have outlived their usefulness. For example, when you were five or six, it was useful to believe that you should not talk to strangers, because they might hurt you. But if you still believe this when you're thirty, it might limit your success in life (and in dating!). Another explanation is that these critical voices are cognitive distortions of reality. Like looking at ourselves in a fun-house mirror, what we see resembles us enough to be familiar, but it doesn't reflect who we actually are.

We love some of the names our clients have come up with for their inner critics: the itty-bitty-shitty committee, the hamster wheel, the evil board of directors, the gang, the naysayer, Mr. Bossypants, Negative Nancy, Aunt Margaret, and many more.

Theorists have also addressed these voices. Jay Earley and Bonnie Weiss have categorized seven types of inner critics: the perfectionist, the taskmaster, the inner controller, the guilt tripper, the destroyer, the underminer, and the molder.[15] Author Richard Carson calls this cast of characters Gremlins.[16] The Coaches Training Institute calls them saboteurs.[17] The Organization and Relationship Systems Coaching model calls them triggered selves.[18] The Inside Team model calls them hijackers.[19]

In addition to our inner critic, let's take a look at three more prominent examples of how negative internal circumstances can cause needless suffering and block us from living *What Matters?!*

COGNITIVE DISTORTIONS

Cognitive distortions are irrational or extreme thoughts that affect one's perception of reality, usually in a negative way. They epitomize negative internal circumstances. Read the following table and ask yourself, do any of these sound familiar? (Not to worry, we have antidotes for you in the next chapter!)

COMMON COGNITIVE DISTORTIONS[20]

DISTORTION	DESCRIPTION
All or Nothing Thinking	Seeing things as black and white, right and wrong, with nothing in between. Essentially, you believe that if you're not perfect, then you're a failure. • "I didn't finish writing that paper, so it was a complete waste of time." • "There's no point in playing if I'm not 100 percent in shape." • "They didn't show; they're completely unreliable."
Over-generalization	Using words like "always" and "never" in relation to a single event or experience. • "I'll never get that promotion." • "She always does that."
Minimizing or Magnifying (aka Catastrophizing)	Seeing things as dramatically more or less important than they actually are, often creating a "catastrophe" that follows. • "Because my boss publicly thanked her, she'll get the promotion, not me (even though I had a great performance review and just won an industry award)." • "I forgot that e-mail! That means my boss won't trust me again, I won't get that raise, and my wife will leave me."
"Shoulds"	Using "should", "need to", "ought to", and "must" to motivate you, then feeling guilty when you don't follow through (or anger and resentment when someone else doesn't follow through). • "I should have gotten the painting done this weekend." • "They ought to have been more considerate of my feelings; they should know that would upset me."
Labeling	Attaching a negative label to yourself or others following a single event. • "I didn't stand up to my coworker. I'm such a wimp!" • "What an idiot, he couldn't even see that coming!"

Mental Filter	Allowing (dwelling on) one negative detail or fact to spoil your enjoyment, happiness, hope, etc. • You have a great evening at a restaurant with friends, but your chicken was undercooked, and that "spoiled the whole night."
Jumping to Conclusions: Mind Reading	Making negative assumptions about how people see you without evidence or factual support. • Your friend is preoccupied and you don't bother to find out why. You're thinking, "She thinks I'm exaggerating again." Or, "He still hasn't forgiven me for telling Fred."
Jumping to Conclusions: Fortune-telling	Making negative predictions about the future without evidence or factual support. • "I won't be able to sell my house and I'll be stuck here." (even though the housing market is good). • "No one will understand. I won't be invited back again." (even though they are supportive friends).
Discounting the Positive	Not acknowledging the positive. Saying anyone could have done it or insisting that your positive actions, qualities, or achievements don't count. • "That doesn't count. Anyone could have done it." • "I've only cut back from smoking forty cigarettes a day to ten. It doesn't count, because I haven't fully quit."
Blame and Personalization	Blaming yourself when you weren't entirely responsible, or blaming other people and denying your role in the situation. • "If only I were younger, I would have gotten the job." • "If only I hadn't said that, they wouldn't have..." • "If only she hadn't yelled at me, I wouldn't have had the car accident."
Emotional Reasoning	I feel, therefore I am. Assuming that a feeling is true without digging deeper to see if it is accurate. • "I feel like such an idiot." (so it must be true). • "I feel guilty." (so I must have done something wrong). • "I feel bad for yelling at my partner." (so I must be selfish and inconsiderate).

If you are someone who is encumbered by inner critics, negative thinking, or cognitive distortions, we invite you to examine them in the following exercise.

WHAT GETS IN THE WAY?

In the left column identify your top three internal circumstances that are interfering with your well-being. In the corresponding right-hand column, record how that particular inner critic, negative thinking, or cognitive distortion is impacting you. Refer to the charts on pages 57, 59, and 60 for examples of internal circumstances.

NEGATIVE THOUGHT, INNER CRITIC, OR COGNITIVE DISTORTION	HOW IT GETS IN THE WAY
e.g., "I've got to get it right!"	Causes me to worry and obsess about projects at my job. Takes me out of being emotionally present with my family on nights and weekends. Prevents me from innovating and taking risks. Sucks the enjoyment out of work.

If all of this talk about negative thinking has got you down, remember, we have some antidotes for you in upcoming chapters!

Irrational Beliefs about Money

You knew it was going to come up sooner or later in a book about *What Matters?!* So here it is: money! If you just felt a stress-induced rush of adrenaline and cortisol, you're not alone. Why? Neuroscientists at the California Institute of Technology have discovered a part of the brain that is responsible for worrying about money.[21] And guess what? Your brain is not at all rational about it. The culprit? Two almond-shaped clusters of tissue called the amygdala, located in the medial temporal lobes. They are part of the brain's limbic system, and they play a primary role in decision-making, emotional reactions, and the processing of memory.

Gallup has even developed a Financial Worry Metric, which found that half of Americans in 2015 suffer from crippling financial anxiety. According to their poll:[22]

- 60 percent of Americans are very/moderately worried about not having enough money for retirement
- 55 percent of Americans are very/moderately worried about not being able to pay medical costs of a serious illness/accident
- 46 percent of Americans are very/moderately worried about not being able to maintain the standard of living they enjoy

Like the rest of the *What Matters?!* framework, your relationship to money is your business, not ours. Our only wish for you is that you don't allow it to hijack your well-being by either causing excessive worry or forcing you to make choices that don't align with who you are.

Take, for example, Joseph, a fifty-year-old single man who has always aspired to own a home. He has a savings of $250,000 and earns $100,000 per year. Every time he finds a suitable property, fear prevents him from making the purchase. He worries, "What if I lose my job? I'd go through my savings and wouldn't have anything to live on when I retire. What if I get sick? How will I pay my medical bills and mortgage?" Our heart goes out to Joseph. What matters to him is owning a home. What also matters is safety and security.

Preoccupation with Past and Future

The fundamental goal of *What Matters?!* is to help you build a firm foundation of strength and calm so that you can live a life of well-being. That's what we call thriving. Thriving occurs now, in this moment. That's not to say we shouldn't spend time learning from the past and planning for the future. However, for many in today's world, the pendulum has swung from a healthy dose of responsible anticipation of the future to excessive worry.

There is a popular saying that is often (and perhaps mistakenly) attributed to ancient Chinese philosopher Lao Tzu. Either way, we still like it!

If you are depressed you are living in the past.
If you are anxious you are living in the future.
If you are at peace you are living in the present.[23]

Other Things that Get in the Way

We could go on and on about what gets in the way of living *What Matters?!* But instead of continuing to focus on the problems, we prefer to move on to the solutions. Before we do, though, here are some additional culprits. We invite you to add your own to the list.

- Need to fit in/conform
- Others' expectations
- Worry/anxiety
- Shame
- Complaining
- Need for immediate gratification
- Sense of obligation
- Need for control
- Being attached to a specific outcome
- Fear of failure
- Defensiveness

As you continue through this book, remember that the goal is to discover the tools that help you mitigate the impact of negative external circumstances by helping you manage your internal circumstances. Mastering your internal circumstances will allow you to make your best choices for creating your optimal future external circumstances.

Laurel's Story: Physician Heal Thyself

Paul spent the other day with a friend of ours and her husband. Our friend is a physician and an accomplished researcher in infectious disease. For years, she has kept up a grueling schedule, but at fifty-years-old, it is finally starting to take its toll. Paul could tell that she wanted to talk.

LAUREL: *Oh no, the new yearly call schedule is coming out. I'm in absolute dread. Every year when this happens, I totally wig out.*

PAUL: *How come?*

LAUREL: *When you are on the call schedule, you basically have to stay up for a week straight. The older I get, and the older the kids get, it's getting more and more difficult to be on-call and to juggle everything else that my boss expects me to do. I used to be able to do it. Now, at fifty-years-old, I just can't do as many call weeks as I used to. By the end of the call week, I can barely function. It's getting so that I'm concerned I might make a mistake out of exhaustion. In fact, last week I snapped at someone when I shouldn't have. I just can't do this again.*

PAUL: *Wow, sounds like you are at a Stop and Ask moment.*

LAUREL: *What do you mean?*

PAUL: *It's one of those times when you realize that what has worked before in your life is no longer working. It's one of those times when it's time to ask yourself what matters and if how you're living aligns with what you say is most important. Mind if I try the* What Matters?! *approach and see where it gets you?*

LAUREL: *Sure. I'll take all the help I can get!*

PAUL: *So, let's start with the basic question. What matters to you?*

LAUREL: *At this point in my life, I definitely have to say my family. I want to be the best possible mom to my kids and be a great partner to my husband. That's not to say that my job isn't extremely important to me. I care a great deal about my patients and want* to find cures for the horrible diseases that they suffer from. But, I have to say family first.

PAUL: Okay, let's start with the first thing you said—your family is most important to you. How are you doing at honoring them, at prioritizing them in your life?

LAUREL: Pretty good. We are very close and spend good quality time together. I think my kids feel safe and loved and my husband feels like we are a good team.

PAUL: Great. So you're living what matters when it comes to your family. Congrats to you! Now, you also said your job matters to you. Let's look there. How are you doing in living what matters when it comes to your job?

LAUREL: Well, that's what started this whole conversation. I'm not.

PAUL: Because . . .

LAUREL: Because of the damn call schedule. It's frying me.

PAUL: Okay, so in the language of the What Matters?! framework, you have an external circumstance, namely the call schedule, that is interfering with your well-being.

LAUREL: What do you mean by an external circumstance?

PAUL: An external circumstance is a condition that exists in the world around you. Some of them you create for yourself, such as having *children or buying a house. Others are created for you, like your age, the call schedule, and infectious diseases.*

LAUREL: *Can I add my crazy boss to that list? How about the budget cuts we are facing? Not to mention my lack of sleep!*

PAUL: *You get the picture. Now, let's take a step back. What matters to you about your job?*

LAUREL: *Well, other than putting food on the table, what matters about my job is caring for people with stigmatized diseases and finding cures.*

PAUL: *If you were living what matters in relation to your job, what would that look like?*

LAUREL: *Ideally, I wouldn't have any call hour weeks.*

PAUL: *Is there any number of call hour weeks that would be acceptable? In other words, an external circumstance that would allow you to live what matters?*

LAUREL: *I could do six call hour weeks in a given year, but no more. That would mean six weeks of little to no sleep.*

PAUL: *So why not sit down with your boss, explain the situation, and request fewer or no call hours?*

LAUREL: *He'll fire me.*

PAUL: *Really? Are you sure?*

LAUREL: *Yup, I've seen it happen before. Three times, in fact.*

PAUL: *Why not have the conversation anyway? If you get fired, you get fired. At least you'll have your sanity, and your patients will get their care from someone who isn't burnt out.*

LAUREL: *I can't get fired.*

PAUL: *Why not?*

LAUREL: *For practical reasons. I'm the one in the family with the steady income and health insurance.*

PAUL: *I see. Health insurance and a steady income are external circumstances that are nonnegotiable.*

LAUREL: *Yes, I told you—family matters. And these are critical components to that.*

PAUL: *Totally get it. Let me ask you something, and really think about it carefully before you answer. Can you be absolutely sure that you'll get fired if you have the conversation?*

LAUREL: *I can't be absolutely sure, but I can't take the risk. Not only do we need the income, but getting fired would blemish my record.*

PAUL: *Okay. Time to talk about internal circumstances. These are beliefs and feelings of your own creation, your reaction to the world around you. The stories you tell yourself that determine your state of mind and the choices you make. In this case, you've created an internal circumstance that it's too risky to talk to your boss. Correct?*

LAUREL: *An internal circumstance that is 99 percent based on reality—a true story as far as any rational person would see it. Might as well be an external circumstance. Just talk to my ex-colleagues who spoke up!*

PAUL: *Okay then, you can't get fired. So, if a steady income and health insurance are the drivers here, why not look for a new job?*

LAUREL: *I could, but all of my colleagues who got fed up and left for other positions have regretted their decision. They thought the grass would be greener and it hasn't been. While they did get back some of their sanity, they miss being on the front line fighting infectious diseases. Plus, how can I know that there is even a position out there where I can do what I want to do?*

PAUL: *Sounds like there's another internal circumstance here. A belief that you won't be able to find a satisfying job.*

LAUREL: *Again, it's a rational conclusion based on data.*

PAUL: *Okay, so let me see if I have this straight. You can speak up about the crazy call hours and risk being fired, or you can find another job and risk having it be unfulfilling. Right?*

LAUREL: *You've got it.*

PAUL: *Any other alternatives?*

LAUREL: *Well, I suppose I could accept the call schedule as published and just know that when I hit the six-week mark, I'm mentally checked out.*

PAUL: *How does that help you?*

LAUREL: *It buys me some time.*

PAUL: *But you'll ultimately either have to talk to your boss or find another job. Correct?*

LAUREL: *Yes.*

PAUL: *So, pay now or pay later.*

LAUREL: *Now that you put it that way . . .*

PAUL: *Okay, here we are back at our Stop and Ask moment. Time for some major truth-telling. You've said your family and job matter. A lot of good you'll be to your husband, your kids, and your patients when you've crashed and burned. So, what's it gonna be?*

LAUREL: *The only thing I'm ready to commit to is having it in my mind that I won't exceed the six weeks. That will allow me to stay present and engaged in my work. Once I hit the six weeks, I'll have to cross that bridge then.*

PAUL: *So you're adjusting your internal circumstances to get you through the short-term. Rather than feeling trapped indefinitely*

*in an untenable situation, you now see yourself temporarily in a
negative external circumstance.*

LAUREL: *It's a story that will keep me sane.*

PAUL: *Laurel, sweetheart, here's where I switch from being a professional
coach to being your friend. You know that's only a Band-Aid, right?*

LAUREL: *I know, but I just can't do anything else right now.*

With that, Paul gave her a hug and wished her well. He was
disappointed that he couldn't talk her into taking a bigger leap
by talking to her boss or looking for a new job. Her internal circumstances simply would not allow it. The good news is, she had
at least found some temporary relief by crafting a new short-term
narrative about the situation.

Two days later Paul received an e-mail message from Laurel's
husband, Barry, which said, "Paul, thank you for coaching Laurel.
In the wake of your discussion, she and I spoke quite a bit more
about what truly matters to us. The conversations have given us
clarity and confidence. To use your language, we've shifted our
internal circumstances from fear of taking risk to the courage to
live what matters. Laurel's health and the well-being of her patients
are paramount. We are no longer willing to tolerate the external
circumstance of the intense call schedule. Bolstered by the power
of that conviction, Laurel had a frank conversation with her boss
yesterday. Holy crap! He actually agreed to limit her to six call
weeks for the coming year! We're still in shock!"

Here's our take (and Laurel confirms it): if there is an external
circumstance that is getting in the way of living what matters, we

owe it to ourselves to dig deep, find our inner truth, and muster the courage to address it, trusting that the outcome—even if negative in the short-term—will ultimately serve us.

Trust that if you're acting on your truth and not hiding out of fear, you will land on your feet and be better for it (although the landing might not always be smooth). Yes, it's a leap of faith, but one worth taking—just ask Laurel.

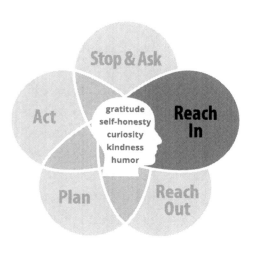

CHAPTER FOUR
REACH IN

Buddhist nun Pema Chödrön wrote, "It has been said that studying ourselves provides all the books we need."[24] In 2012, Paul experienced the truth of that statement when he underwent emergency neck surgery. Unable to work, he lay on the couch immobilized, cloaked with unease about going back to professional life as he knew it. A midlife crisis? A longing for something different? It was time to Stop and Ask.

Over the next few months, Paul readied himself for a much-needed Thoreau-esque sabbatical. With David's support, he jettisoned all of his remaining work responsibilities and went to live in a 300-square-foot cottage on the tip of Cape Cod in Provincetown, a place with a long history of welcoming those in need of soul searching. Brando the dog came along for companionship.

For the next three months, Paul lived an unstructured life dedicated to going to "the school of me." Daily journaling, bike rides, walks in nature, kayaking, gardening—he even stepped outside of his comfort zone and took a painting class. All of this had him connecting with himself in ways that he never had before. Paul was fortunate that he could take three months for reflection, exploration, and reconnecting with his heart. When we pause to Reach In, it doesn't need to be for three months. It can also be for three days, three hours, or three minutes. Regardless of the length of time, there are a variety of tools that can help you reclaim your well-being and toss out what is getting in the way.

RESILIENCY

The goal of the *What Matters?!* framework is to increase your overall well-being. A key component of the practices and mindsets is to build up your personal resiliency. Personal resiliency is about managing the people, thoughts, and things that can cause you stress—those external circumstances discussed in the last chapter. Although you may not be able to change any of them, you *can* change how you relate to them and react to them. It is our hope that Reaching In will become second nature to you so that you can build up your resiliency reserves.

If your life isn't working for you, you owe it to yourself to Reach In and explore alternative ways of living.

The path you choose to take may not be what you or others expected, since you, your family, your friends, and society all bombard you with subtle and not-so-subtle messages about what life should look like. When Paul first got into coaching, friends would ask what it entailed. David would say, "Paul helps you figure out what you wanted to do with your life before your parents and society beat it out of you."

BODY, MIND, AND SPIRIT

So, you've Stopped and Asked. Like many people, you have probably found areas where you are not honoring what matters to you. Now what? Time to Reach In and realign your body, mind, and spirit.

BODY

When we look at our bodies, we have to ask ourselves, What are we doing to take care of the beautiful—yes, we said beautiful—bodies that we have? (And if you don't think your body is beautiful, we will address that shortly when we talk about working with our inner critic.)

WORKING IT

We invite you to Reach In and reflect on the following questions:
- ✓ Are you feeding your body the best food possible?
- ✓ Are you exercising regularly?
- ✓ Are you getting quality sleep every night?
- ✓ Are you limiting or eliminating harmful physical influences (alcohol, tobacco, recreational drugs)?

PHYSICAL HEALTH INVENTORY

1. When was your last physical exam?

2. When was your last dental exam?

3. When was your last eye exam?

4. How many times per week do you exercise?

5. Do you walk or bike when you can, as opposed to driving?

6. Do you get at least seven hours of sleep per night?

7. How much alcohol do you consume? Sugar? Caffeine?

8. What are your eating habits? Do you eat breakfast every day?

9. Do you drink at least eight glasses of water per day?

Many of the warning signs that a Stop and Ask is needed—what we call a What Matters?! Red Alert—manifest as physical symptoms of discomfort: trouble sleeping, body aches, headaches, weight gain, weight loss. Of course, sometimes a Red Alert can manifest emotionally: unresolvable anger, chronic sadness, or even lack of emotion, numbness. It can also manifest as unexplainable health problems or stress-related illnesses, like ulcers, irritable bowel syndrome, and chronic fatigue.

If our exercise reads like one of those checklists at the doctor's office, it was meant to. Plenty of research proves there's a direct connection between too much stress and poor physical and mental health. When we're in Red Alert, we're in a state where we've been ignoring for a long time what matters to us, and our bodies are often the first warning we hear—or the last one we can no longer avoid.

LISA M.'S STORY: CHOOSING HEALTH

Lisa M., one of our What Matters?! Workshop attendees, had spent a lifetime battling her weight and had tried everything out there to combat it—counting calories, following traditional weight loss plans, and enlisting personal trainers. Finally, she decided it was time to take matters into her own hands. She Stopped and Asked herself what was holding her back and whether or not all of these attempts at health had actually worked. They hadn't.

Her weight was at an all-time high. She had joint and back pain, her cholesterol and blood pressure were through the roof, travel had become difficult, and she could not live the active life she had always wanted. In short, she was miserable, and everyone around her knew it.

She Reached In and evaluated how she felt about herself and what she could do to improve her feelings of self-worth. She spent time identifying the positives about herself that were not dependent on her weight. Finally, she spent time unraveling all of the put-downs she had told herself based on her appearance.

After spending time thinking about her potential next steps, Lisa Reached Out and talked to people in similar situations. Then she spent months Planning—researching and investigating the pros and cons of her options. She started following a medically monitored low-calorie diet. She lost two pounds in two months and became discouraged.

Finally, Lisa met with a bariatric surgeon. "You know what your problem is?" he asked. "You're not seven feet tall." They both laughed, and Lisa knew this was the right choice to Act on. She began the long, arduous process of preparing for surgery and life afterward: doctor appointments, medical approvals, and attending group workshops.

When she was wheeled into the operating room, she was confident that this would be one of her best life decisions. Despite her fears, she had chosen to Act on what was right for her. In the last two years, she has lost over one hundred pounds, seven dress sizes, and several inches around her waist.

She can now be found running 5Ks, traveling frequently, writing about her experiences, and motivating others to discover What Matters?!

MIND

In the last chapter we painted quite a bleak picture of how our thoughts can create needless suffering. Here we would like to offer you some new perspectives and tools for navigating the sometimes dangerous neighborhood of our minds.

Thinking a thought and believing a thought are two very different things.

How many times have you been on an airplane and the thought has suddenly occurred to you that the plane could go down? It's just a thought. The trouble begins when you actually start believing it. (We apologize if you happen to be reading this while on a plane. Breathe.) So, even if you've assumed your inner critics, cognitive distortions, and other negative thoughts were true for most of your life, they still only have power because you *believe* them.

You may have even gathered lots of evidence to prove that your negative thoughts are true. But evidence-gathering is highly subjective. A well-known term in psychology and sociology is *confirmation bias*. It's defined by social psychologist Scott Plous as "the tendency to search for, interpret, favor, and recall information in a way that confirms one's beliefs or hypotheses, while giving disproportionately less consideration to alternative possibilities."[25] In other words, we focus on certain parts of our experience or environment and ignore others. If you've ever noticed that you pay more attention to subtle criticism than to clear, direct compliments, you know what we're talking about.

NAVIGATING THE NEIGHBORHOOD OF YOUR MIND

Ever tried to silence the negative thoughts by willing them to stop or by trying to push them out of your mind? Psychologists call this *thought stopping*, and it's definitely not one of our favorite techniques. In fact, thought stopping is more likely to lead to *thought rebounding*. In the words of Carl Jung, "What you resist persists."[26]

Author and teacher Byron Katie explains, "We can't *stop* thinking about a stressful thought. We have to examine it, and get to the truth behind our stories. Then and only then, when we no longer believe the thought, the thought lets go of us."[27]

Katie's model, called The Work (www.thework.com), takes any thought or story that causes distress and asks, "Is it true?" Then it steps through a simple process to turn that story around, so that the negative thought dissolves and is replaced with one that is useful.

There are many other Reach In mind tools out there, which should tell you how common it is to be hobbled by negative thinking. Here are some of our favorites.

- Rick Carson's book *Taming Your Gremlin* offers a number of approaches for personifying your inner critics' voices and neutralizing their impact through a series of playful exercises.[28]
- Organization and Relationship Systems Coaching, created by Faith Fuller and Marita Fridjhon of the Center for Right Relationship (crrglobal.com), offers a detriggering process to separate your inner critics from your core self and diffuse their power.
- The concept of mindfulness—taught everywhere from meditation programs to corporate effectiveness classes—helps you be present and aware of what's happening in the moment, without judging.
- Julia Cameron in her book *The Artist's Way* shares a practice she calls "morning pages"—you write three pages in longhand by stream of consciousness first thing in the morning.[29] Paul

practices a form of this Reach In every day. Putting thoughts on paper rather than letting them clog your head is the first step to a centered, engaging day.

• Acceptance and Commitment Therapy includes a method called diffusion, which is learning to see thoughts and feelings for what they are—streams of words, passing sensations, or emotions—rather than what they claim to be—dangers or facts. Check out Russ Harris's *The Happiness Trap*.[30] It has a wealth of tools for rescuing your mind from uncomfortable thoughts and feelings.

YOUR INNER TEAM

Before we give the mind too bad a rap, we want to point out that not all of your inner voices are negative. They are simply members of a larger club that we call your *inner team*, also known by many as your *internal board of directors*. Like any board of directors, there certainly are those negative voices, like the ones we pointed out in the last chapter. However—and here's the good news—your board also has allies, those voices that encourage and support you: your cheerleader, your optimist, your adventurer. You can look inside and find your own names for them.

Are you having a hard time hearing the positive voices over the bedlam of the negative ones? Think about the people who believe in you or believed in you. What positive icons can you mentally call upon? The dreamer? The bulldozer? The wise owl? Whoever or whatever they are, make sure that they have a seat at your boardroom table. You might even want one of them to sit at the head.

As our dear friend and exceptional coach Beth Shapiro often tells clients, we must choose what aspects of ourselves to pay attention to. Imagine that your thoughts are a garden of sun-loving plants. The ones you shine the light on are the ones that will grow. Your attention is the light. Spend lots of attention listening to, or even arguing with, your inner critic and it will get stronger. Focus your attention instead on your positive voices, and they will grow stronger, too.

And if the critical, anxious, scared, and other so-called "negative" members of your inner team just won't quiet down, here's another perspective that you may want to consider. What if, in fact, they are not intentionally trying to derail you but just tend to have the loudest voices because they are trying to protect you from perceived danger? Don't push them away. They'll come back stronger than ever. Instead, talk to them openly and constructively. The following tool will help you.

YOUR INNER TEAM

1. Identify the members of your inner team who are causing you discomfort.

2. Complete one of the following worksheets for each inner team member. Listen with curiosity about what they are trying to tell you. Use the questions on the worksheet to see how you can turn their concerns into something that will serve you rather than scare you.

3. If you choose, write worksheets for the more positive members of your inner team as a way to leverage the encouragement and strengths they provide.

NAME OF INNER TEAM MEMBER: _____

a) What important thing (safety, success, etc.) does this team member want for you in relationship to the issue you are struggling with?

b) What do you appreciate about the team member in relationship to this issue?

c) What do you want more of from this team member in relationship to this issue?

d) What do you want less of from this team member in relationship to this issue?

e) How can this team member be of greater assistance in helping you to live your most fulfilling life?

WHERE DO VALUES FIT INTO THE EQUATION?

If inner critics are the negative parts of our inner world, our values are our inner world at its best. Leadership expert Stan Slap says, "Values are deeply held personal beliefs that form your own priority code for living. . . . They're the definition of what life looks like when you live it exactly the way you want to."[31] In other words, when you pay attention to what matters to you, you are moving closer to your values.

There is a strong link between well-being and values. Kelly Wilson, a pioneer in Acceptance and Commitment Therapy, says, "The scientific evidence strongly suggests that active engagement with your values builds strength." He cites the research of J. D. Creswell, who "showed that under stressful situations, people who are more engaged with their values produce lower levels of cortisol, a neurotransmitter that over the long-term makes people less resilient and more prone to mental and physical illness."[32]

Before *What Matters?!* David developed affordable housing in Boston. One development he was working on had many competing stakeholders—one of the groups was particularly contentious and bullied people into getting its way. David was preparing for a meeting with about twenty people from this group who wanted some concessions that would hurt other community groups. David would be representing the developer, and the meeting would be attended by several city, state, and federal government representatives. Prior to the meeting, David was nervous and voiced his concerns to one of his favorite mentors, Michael Groden. After listening to David, Mike said matter-of-factly, "What have you got to be worried about? As long as you are 'in the right,' you have nothing to be nervous about."

This was the shift in view David needed. He realized he had nothing to fear, because he was doing what was right for the development and all of the other concerned parties. He was honoring his values of fairness and social justice. This particular group was overreaching with their demands. In fact, the reason they were being bullies was precisely because they were not acting in good faith. The outcome of the meeting was a fair distribution of concessions for all parties. David was no longer afraid, he was empowered—and that's a lesson he holds to this day.

How do you know what your values are? Think about what energizes you, like connecting with friends or presenting your research. Or you might recognize your values based on what angers you, like finding out a friend has lied. You may feel centered when you are working on things that express your values, like precise analysis or wild creativity. Or you might feel off-kilter when you're doing things that don't, like spending long hours inside when you love the outdoors. Interested in exploring your values? Try the following exercise.

WORKING IT

Here's a simple way to uncover your values. Think back to a time when you felt fully alive, engaged, awake, and present. It doesn't necessarily have to be a fun time. For example, you might have felt fully alive while giving birth, which probably wasn't too much fun; or you might have been very present while sitting with a dying friend.

When you've identified the memory, write a quick, simple description of it. Don't worry about grammar or spelling, you can even just make a list of words or short phrases. Include details such as what you were doing; who you were with; where you were; what the weather was like; how things smelled, tasted, felt. What was meaningful about it to you? What moment really stands out? Now look at what you wrote down. Circle the words that express what was most important about the experience. Congratulations. You've just identified some of your core values.

It's important not just to know your values, but to live them. Imagine that you are a lightbulb on a dimmer switch. When you choose activities that express your values, you have a stronger power source and your brightness increases. When you choose to act on the advice of your inner critic—to re-act according to your inner critic's beliefs—you cut yourself off from your power source, and you shed less light, and thus, see things less clearly.

Spirit

Recall Laura Whitworth's warning to Paul in chapter 3: don't visit the dangerous neighborhood of your mind alone. If we aren't supposed to go alone, who should we go with? The Reach Out practice, which is coming up soon, clearly shows that we live best when we ask for help and support from our fellow humans. But what about resources that transcend human intervention? Just like everything else in this book, this section on spirit is an invitation, one for you to think about. If it resonates, that's wonderful; if it doesn't, that's cool, too. We simply invite you to explore this area.

For us personally, spirit is one of our favorite areas, one that we are constantly learning about. Spirit can be brought into every facet of our lives—it is the secret sauce of life. There are many definitions of spirit; but for us, spirit is about feeling less isolated and alone in the world by living the best we can with open and caring hearts.

For those looking for a textbook definition, here is one from Dr. Ruth Murray and Judith Zentner, authors of *Health Promotion Strategies through the Life Span*: "Spirituality is a quality that goes beyond religious affiliation, that strives for inspiration, reverence, awe, meaning and purpose, even in those who do not believe in God."[33]

For some people, spirit may take the form of organized religion, which will be discussed in Reach Out. For the purposes of Reach In, we discuss spirit as our unique relationship with what is greater than ourselves. You can use the term *spirit, heart, soul, higher power, nature, passion,* or whatever fits best for you.

WORKING IT

✓ How important to you is spirit/spirituality?
✓ What is your definition of spirit/spirituality?
✓ To what extent is spirit/spirituality present in your life?
✓ What do you do to connect with "spirit"?
✓ What would be possible in your life by strengthening your spirit/spirituality?

THE WISDOM TO KNOW THE DIFFERENCE

As we close our discussion of Reach In, we reiterate the distinction between internal and external circumstances. Internal circumstances are our thoughts and beliefs, most notably our *negative* thoughts and beliefs that swirl around in our head and keep us from living a life of well-being. External circumstances are situations many of which are beyond our control. For those that are negative and out of our control, we can learn Reach In tools and techniques to help us manage their adverse impact. For those negative external circumstances in our control we can act to change the circumstances themselves. But how to know when a circumstance is in or out of our control?

One of our favorite Reach In tools is the Serenity Prayer, which says, "God, grant me the serenity to accept the things I cannot change, the courage to change the things I can, and the wisdom to know the difference." The majority of twelve-step program meetings conclude with this prayer. It is a common misconception that this prayer originated in Alcoholics Anonymous. In fact, it was authored by American theologian Reinhold Niebuhr in the 1930s. Its message resonated with AA's cofounders and they wove it into the fabric of their program. It resonates for us as well, so much so that we have incorporated its premise into our *What Matters?!* planning tool, which we'll introduce in chapter 8.

In order to live *What Matters?!*, you will need to Reach In—do whatever it takes to get in clear, grounded alignment with your body, mind, and spirit. The tools we use to Reach In nourish us and build up our resiliency to handle current and future circumstances. Examples of Reaching In can be as simple as eating a good meal, walking, dancing, journaling, listening to music, meditation, or prayer. Whatever works for you, works! It's about you being at your best, calling forth your strength and facing every circumstance from a place of choice.

WORKING IT

The following table offers some more examples of ways you can Reach In.

✓ Place a checkmark by those examples that resonate with you.
✓ Place an asterisk next to those that are new for you and you might want to try.
✓ Identify at least one Reach In practice that you will do this week.

BODY	MIND	SPIRIT
Yoga	Write in a journal	Be in nature
Pilates	Meditate	Sing
Eat healthy foods	Use cognitive reframing tools found in books such as:	Paint/draw
Dance		Read something that inspires you
Bike	Loving What Is	Visit a hospital or nursing home
Jog	The Happiness Trap	
Lift weights	Identify and question your go-to cognitive distortions (see pages 59 & 60)	Volunteer
Walk		Play an instrument
Stretch		Read to a child
Drink water	Practice self-compassion using tools such as those found on www.self-compassion.org	Pat your pet
Keep a food diary		Listen to music
	Conduct a "meeting" of your "inner team." (see page 85)	Think about what you are grateful for
	Knit	Do something kind for someone
	Be curious	

I commit to doing the following Reach In practice this week:

_____

KAREN'S STORY: STAY OR GO? A MARITAL STRUGGLE

Karen attended one of our What Matters?! workshops and she eventually became one of our clients. Karen's impetus for *exploring What Matters?! was concern for her marriage. She had been married to Peter for twenty-five years, and they had a twenty-three-year-old daughter, who was successfully on her own, as well as a son, who was a sophomore in high school and was finally thriving after several difficult years.*

For the past seven years, Peter had struggled with a chronic heart problem, but in the past several months, he had reached the brink of frustration and had become emotionally and verbally abusive to Karen. At first he was judgmental, then his words turned into ridicule, at first in private, then in front of the children, and eventually in front of friends on social occasions. Karen talked to Peter about it, but he insisted that he was doing nothing wrong. Karen's family and friends had often commented on Peter's controlling behavior. For years he had demanded—and Karen had abided—that what happened behind their four walls was nobody else's business.

Although Karen had thought about leaving Peter, she said to herself, "How could I leave a sick man?" Actually, her initial thought was, "What would people think of me if I left a sick man?" It wasn't until Karen began confiding in her siblings that she realized she was in an abusive relationship. Although Karen's siblings had a good relationship with Peter, they had each thought something was amiss at home. Now with Peter even more frustrated, they feared that his emotional and verbal abuse could turn physical.

Karen's siblings and friends urged her to talk to an attorney. They also helped her brainstorm both a short- and long-term plan as well as an emergency plan.

Karen asked Peter to go to marriage counseling, but he refused. She decided that regardless of his choice, she needed to see a therapist to help her sort through her feelings. Both Peter and Karen were active members of their parish, so Karen Reached Out to their parish priest, who was well-respected in the community and whom she and Peter were fond of. Much to her surprise, Father Tony told her that she did not owe Peter anything, that she had been an incredibly supportive and loving wife. He said that Peter's current actions and treatment were not in keeping with the church's teachings or their marital vows and that she had no obligation to stay with him.

Karen felt a great sense of relief, like she had gotten permission to leave. Now the Stop and Ask question was, What did she really want to do? Stay or go? Her biggest concern was her teenage son—she wasn't sure what was best for him.

She Reached In and asked herself what mattered to her at this point in her life. She contemplated getting an apartment, as her family and friends had urged her, but she decided instead that she would create her own life within her existing circumstances. Yes, she could have left, and perhaps she could have taken her son with her, but she decided that staying at home until he was in college was the least disruptive choice. Providing a stable home life for her son was what mattered most to Karen, something she valued above everything else.

Life was not going to continue as it had previously, however. Karen was going to live on her terms. With this major shift in her thinking, the situation suddenly became more tolerable. When Peter started to ridicule her, she simply left the room. She moved out of their bedroom into the guest room and she started planning activities on the weekend that involved her family and friends.

She continued her coaching sessions and her therapy, she started doing Pilates, and she even went out-of-state to visit her sister—something that had previously been unthinkable since Peter had required all trips to be taken together (otherwise how would it look?).

Karen continued inviting Peter to therapy, and he continued to refuse. She became more independent and confident as she kept on with her self-care. Her family and friends commented on her palpable change, saying that the "old Karen" was back.

Whether it was seeing his wife flourish or his fear that she was doing better without him, Peter eventually went to counseling. With the help of the therapist, Karen had a safe environment to call out Peter's behavior, and she realized that Peter did not have the self-awareness to know that he had been wrong. Slowly, Peter saw how damaging his words and actions could be. And Karen realized that she was guilty of sometimes purposefully triggering his behavior. Together they learned tools for having What Matters?! conversations and things started to improve.

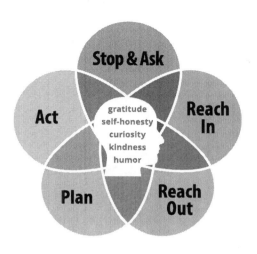

CHAPTER FIVE
THE FIVE MINDSETS

So far we have looked at two of the five *What Matters?!* practices: 1) Stop and Ask and 2) Reach In. In the *What Matters?!* language, *practices* are intentional behavioral habits that enhance well-being—or in other words, the "doing" of the framework. Before we continue with the other three *What Matters?!* practices, let's pause to more thoroughly explore another key component of the *What Matters?!* framework: the five *mindsets*.

As we mentioned in chapter 2, the *What Matters?!* mindsets form the basis of how we experience the world around us. Backed by research from the field of positive psychology, these five mindsets are a universal set of internal circumstances proven to enhance well-being.

In other words, if the practices on their own are the engine, then these mindsets are the fuel—and as simple as they are, we think they are rocket fuel. When you view life through the lenses of humor, kindness, self-honesty, curiosity, and gratitude, you can't help but be less reactive to your external circumstances, which in turn allows you to mindfully choose and boost your well-being. These lenses, however, are not rose-colored—far from it! They are conscious ways of living that will elevate mood, restore motivation, and encourage us to live *What Matters?!*

HUMOR

Lighten up. Life is better when you don't take everything— including *What Matters?!*—so damn seriously. Relax and have a laugh, even at your own expense.

By injecting humor into your daily routine and poking some fun at yourself, you can elevate mood and increase your well-being, self-esteem, resilience, hope, optimism, energy, and vigor while reducing depression, anxiety, and tension.

Still don't think there is anything serious about humor? Actually, the emotional and physical benefits of humor have been well-documented. A University of Maryland study found that a sense of humor can protect against heart disease.[34] Additionally, Gurinder S. Bains, a PhD candidate at Loma Linda University, says, "As an older adult, you will face age-associated memory deficits, but humor and laughter can be integrated into a whole person wellness plan that can translate into improvements in your quality of life: mind, body, and spirit."[35]

But wait, there's even more evidence that humor isn't just a laughing matter. The 2010 PBS television series "This Emotional Life" reveals the following physical benefits of humor: increased endorphins and dopamine, increased relaxation response, reduced pain, and reduced stress. The show also demonstrates humor's cognitive benefits: increased creativity, problem-solving, and an ability to cope with stress. Hey, you employers out there, there's your business case for lightening up!

HUMOR IN ACTION

Our friend Jack moved his mother into his home to care for her as her Alzheimer's progressed. A few months into the new living situation, David asked how it was going and Jack said, "On the worst days I think of how my landlord would react if he knew how many people my mother imagined lived in this apartment."

WORKING IT

Don't think you have a funny bone? No worries, here are some techniques for cultivating a sense of humor.

✓ Laughter is contagious. See a funny movie, go to the circus, or invite friends over to watch "I Love Lucy."
✓ Find at least one situation to laugh at during your day (but please, not at someone else's expense—see the next mindset of Kindness).
✓ Check out a New Yorker cartoon or Dilbert's latest debacle.
✓ Turn your anxieties and fears into funny stories about yourself.
✓ Take an improv comedy class.

KINDNESS

Be kind, for everyone you meet is fighting a battle
you know nothing about.

—WENDY MASS, BEST-SELLING AUTHOR

What is kindness, and how do we apply it to the *What Matters?!* process? You can think of kindness simply as leading with your heart or approaching situations with an open heart. This doesn't mean you're naïve or uninformed; rather, you're mindfully choosing to view a situation through a certain lens.

We are all wired differently, and for some, kindness comes easily. These people tend to lead with their hearts and be more naturally empathetic. Others lead with their heads and are more rational. To be authentically kind, however, we must learn to feel through our hearts.

In the *What Matters?!* framework, kindness includes kindness to self. In fact, for each of us to achieve sustainable well-being, that is where kindness needs to start. People who score high on tests of self-compassion (people who view themselves kindly) have less depression and anxiety, and tend to be happier and more optimistic.

David R. Hamilton is a chemist who left a career developing cardiac and cancer drugs to study the health benefits of kindness and happiness. He's found that acting kindly increases our dopamine, the "feel good" neurotransmitter that is the brain's natural equivalent of morphine and heroin.[36] The result? A "helper's high," so named by Allan Luks and Peggy Payne in their book, *The Healing Power of Doing Good.*[37]

Dr. Hamilton also found that kindness actually slows the aging process. Two factors that contribute to aging are free radicals and inflammation in the cardiovascular system; the hormone oxytocin counteracts the damage from these two. And yep, you guessed it—kindness produces oxytocin. Imagine, kindness is the fountain of youth we've all been seeking!

KINDNESS IN ACTION

Our friend Chris recently posted this on Facebook:

> *OMG. I got in a car accident 2 weeks ago and the lady just sent me a THANK YOU note and a gift card! She slammed into*

my truck hitch. Me, not a scratch but she had damage and her radiator was leaking all over.

She was really upset and apologizing profusely. I got out and gave her a big hug. Made sure she was ok and calmed her down. She was surprised I was being so nice. I told her. I am a cancer survivor. Every day is a gift. My uncle died last week and my aunt died last night. Cars can be replaced but people can't. I waited for the police and tow truck, gave her my biz card and told her if she ever needed window treatments to give me a call! We hugged again and said goodbye. I got this in the mail today! Moral of the story. Be good to people. It always comes back to you!

In her note, the woman had written, "Thank you for being so kind to me on the day of my accident. If there were more people like you, this world would be a better place."

Working It

Want to develop your kindness muscles? Give these a shot:

- ✓ Leave money in a tip jar when the person you're tipping isn't looking (giving without the need for acknowledgement is the purest expression of kindness).
- ✓ When someone is rude or disrespectful, ask yourself, What must it be like to live in his or her mind?
- ✓ Envision how your favorite hero of peace would respond to a situation (e.g., Dalai Lama, the Pope, Gandhi, Mother Teresa, Martin Luther King Jr.).
- ✓ Allow someone to jump ahead of you in line.
- ✓ Visit www.choosetobenice.com and sign the kindness pledge.
- ✓ Visit Dr. Kristen Neff's website at http://self-compassion.org to help you build your self-compassion muscles and stop beating yourself up.

SELF-HONESTY

Throughout the book we have been advocating replacing your thoughts of *should*, *shouldn't*, *have to*, and *can't* with what is really true for you. The self-honesty mindset requires that you embrace and act on the knowledge you receive, even if it doesn't align with others' expectations.

When we first showed the *What Matters?!* framework to our inner circle, a number of them questioned our use of the term *self-honesty*. "Isn't honesty just plain honesty?" Here's the difference.

The essence of *What Matters?!* is knowing what is true for you—likes, dislikes, values, beliefs—and making choices that honor these deepest parts of who you are. Shakespeare's Polonius was an early teacher of *What Matters?!* "This above all: to thine own self be true."

Only you can truly know what matters to you, what makes you come alive and feel good about your life. Your parents can't tell you. Your spouse can't tell you. Your clergy can't tell you. Your friends can't tell you. Only you really know.

Self-honesty is telling the truth about yourself *to yourself*, even if that truth is uncomfortable. We all see ourselves in a certain way, based on how the people around us tell us we should be and how *we* think we should be.

You might be used to looking in the mirror and saying, "I'm a lawyer. I've trained to be a lawyer, I have experience being a lawyer.

I'm good at being a lawyer, I've always seen myself as a lawyer. What's more, my father always wanted me to be a lawyer." This is what you think your identity is. It's familiar and known. But the day might come when you realize you are not all that happy being a lawyer. Then, when you look in the mirror with self-honesty, you suddenly see something else. You see that even though "lawyer" has long been your identity, it's not what you want to be doing. You see that it no longer reflects what matters to you. You might even see that it never really did.

So what now? Suppose you are that lawyer, and you have two kids heading to college, and you have that house in an affluent suburb and a fancy car and a spouse with a penchant for nice things.

Then you need to practice even more self-honesty. You might decide that putting your kids through college is what matters most to you and that you don't have the energy or other resources to leave your job right now. Or you might decide that your kids can shoulder some of the cost of college through loans or scholarships, and so you can afford to make some changes. Or you might realize that you are so stressed and miserable at your job that you have become a total tyrant around the house, and if you stay at that job, you'll actually be hurting your family.

It's up to you to be honest with yourself about what really matters, but you also have to consider your current responsibilities and the impact on those who count on you.

One other important note about self-honesty. This concept comes to us from twelve-step programs, where you must be honest with yourself about your addiction and the damage it's causing to you and those around you. *What Matters?!* is about personal choices that increase our well-being and decrease our suffering. When we can't see the harm our choices are causing, to ourselves or others, we need self-honesty and we need to reach out for help. If people say you have a drug problem, for example, they are concerned about you. Same thing if people are saying you look stressed or that you seem to always have a health problem or you need to come up for air. Look in the mirror and ask what they might be trying to help you see.

Self-honesty is, in part, about paying attention to cues and signals—from your inner self, from those around you, and from that mysterious place often called the universe.

SELF-HONESTY IN ACTION

Health and fitness guru Jenn Menzer has a great line when you're feeling tempted by treats: "They are cute to look at and yummy to eat, too, but probably not fun to wear." That's a combination of humor and self-honesty to help you stay on your healthy eating goals.

WORKING IT

Ready to be truly honest with yourself? Ask yourself the following questions:

- ✓ What is it that I'm afraid to admit to myself?
- ✓ What am I merely tolerating in my life?
- ✓ What are my behaviors and habits that do not serve me?
- ✓ What are the "shoulds" that are sucking the life out of me?
- ✓ What do I need to do to take better care of me?

CURIOSITY

With the curiosity mindset, you open up opportunities. You discover the possibilities inherent in any situation by looking at it with fresh perspective and seeing what can be, which explains why studies have shown that curiosity positively correlates with intelligence.[39]

Renowned positive psychologists Martin Seligman and Chris Peterson have identified and described the top twenty-four human strengths. Among these strengths, curiosity is "one of the five most highly associated strengths for overall life fulfillment and happiness."[40]

Remember the old proverb "curiosity killed the cat?" Well, for us humans, curiosity actually has the exact opposite effect. A 1996 article in *Psychology and Aging* detailed a study of more than one thousand older adults aged fifty to eighty-six over a five-year period. Those who were rated as more curious at the beginning of the study were more likely to be alive at its conclusion, even after taking into account age, smoking habits, and the presence of cancer or cardiovascular disease.[41] Other studies report that curiosity decreases the risk of hypertension and diabetes.

CURIOSITY IN ACTION

To see curiosity in action, let's use one of our favorite examples of emotional hijacking: road rage. Imagine you are driving down the highway and someone cuts in front of you with a move you deem to be reckless and dangerous. Immediately adrenaline and cortisol surge through your body and you think, "That idiot almost killed me."

Now imagine mentally stopping yourself and injecting curiosity into the situation. You might think, "Wow, I wonder what is going on in his life? Maybe he's driving like that because his wife was just rushed to the hospital. Poor guy. I hope his wife is okay." When you choose curiosity, you not only prevent an emotional hijacking, you also develop empathy for the other driver and gratitude that you are not in such a state. In the end, you save yourself from feeling agitated and aggressive, which only harms you—it doesn't affect the other driver one way or the other. Remember, this is about your well-being. Be good to yourself.

WORKING IT

Practice makes progress. Give these curiosity tools a try:

✓ View your situation through the eyes of a seven-year-old.
✓ Ask someone what matters to them.
✓ Have a conversation with someone where you only ask questions.
✓ Ask yourself, "What's it like to live inside that person's head?"
✓ Find the "unfamiliar" in the "familiar."

GRATITUDE

Gratitude is taking the time to be thankful for the gifts in your life. People who are grateful are happier, and the best part is, increasing your gratitude is completely within your control.

You don't have to look far to find things to be grateful for; in fact, if you are reading this book, you should be grateful for the ability to read— how often do we reflect on that? Often we get caught up in wanting and wishing ("Boy, I'd love to have a [vacation, second home, boat]") rather than appreciating the many things we do have.

Robert Emmons, the world's leading scientific expert on gratitude, found that people who practice gratitude consistently report a host of benefits. Physically, they have stronger immune systems, are less bothered by aches and pains, have lower blood pressure, exercise more, take better care of their health, sleep longer, and feel more refreshed upon waking. Psychologically, they experience and exhibit more positive emotions, such as joy and pleasure, optimism and happiness, and they are more alert, alive, and awake. Socially, they are more helpful, generous, compassionate, forgiving, and outgoing, and they feel less lonely and isolated.[42]

According to the Greater Good Science Center at the University of California-Berkeley, "Research suggests these benefits are available to most anyone who practices gratitude, even in the midst of adversity, such as elderly people confronting death, women with breast cancer, and people coping with a chronic muscular disease."[43]

The wonderful power of gratitude is that it can change your mood or perspective instantly. Our dear friend and favorite optimist, Andrea, has three teenage daughters and is helping them build their lives with integrity, grace, and humor. As is the case when you have even the most wonderful children, there are bad days. One Monday morning, all three girls had a definite tone of crankiness, to which Andrea exclaimed, "Change your attitude! Start with gratitude!" Then she asked each of the girls to name one thing they were thankful for. With each response, the mood brightened, and the girls left for school with a new, positive outlook.

GRATITUDE IN ACTION

David was sitting in an aisle seat on a packed flight from Boston to Chicago. Seated next to him in the middle seat was a ten-year-old boy, Jack, and next to him in the window seat was his mother, Judy. Judy told David that Jack was severely autistic, and she apologized in advance for any inconvenience it may cause during the flight.

David had little experience with autistic children and was unsure of what to expect from this boy who would be confined to a seat for three hours. David Reached In and asked for some spiritual guidance. The answer that came was gratitude. As David witnessed Jack have many outbursts over the next three hours, he was amazed at the love, compassion, and patience that Judy had for her son. She would talk to him in a soft voice and stroke him; he would calm down and feel more comfortable in his own skin (that was how Judy described it). David was on the plane for three hours, but this was Judy's life. David said a little prayer, thanking God for having given this special boy such an amazing mother. What could have been a frustrating situation turned into a beautiful experience of appreciation.

Working It

Want to strengthen your attitude of gratitude? Here are some suggestions:

- ✓ At night and/or in the morning, identify three things for which you are grateful. Write them down in a journal or put them on scraps of paper in a jar.
- ✓ During dinner, invite each family member to share something for which they are grateful. Conduct a round robin and see how many times you can make it around the table.
- ✓ Sit in the lobby of a children's hospital.
- ✓ Spend the day in a wheelchair.
- ✓ Volunteer at a soup kitchen.

As you go forward practicing the *What Matters?!* approach, remember that in addition to the "doing" of the practices, it is important to incorporate the "being" of the five mindsets. The goal is to decrease stress in your life and increase your well-being. Sometimes simply looking through a different lens is all it takes to shift how you think and react to a situation. What's simple, though, is not always easy. It may not be easy to stop and figure out a new perspective, but it can make all the difference. And you may have to try on more than one of the mindsets to shift your thinking.

A bonus of using these mindsets is that they not only help your well-being, they also tend to help the well-being of everyone around you!

LISA S.'S STORY: A HARD LOOK IN THE MIRROR LEADS TO LOVE

Lisa has an upbeat, bubbly personality. She is fun to be around, the kind of friend you can call on for anything. Unfortunately, she had fallen into a "bad dating rut," going through a series of boyfriends who were not good to her or good for her. In her middle thirties, with most of her friends married and having children, she had convinced herself that she was lucky to be dating any guy she could get.

Quick interjection here: Have you ever been telling a friend about a challenge you're facing, and as you are describing the situation, you realize how completely crazy it sounds? Now see what Lisa had to say in her own words.

Tim, who I was dating, moved into my apartment not because we were ready to move to the next level in our relationship, but because his previous apartment had been sold. He was a slick salesman and a cheapskate to boot. He played off of my insecurities and convinced me that he was a catch. Although my rent was $1,200/month, he was only paying me $400/month, because that is what his share of his old apartment was. As he put it, it was

$400 more a month than I was getting before! He was so cheap he would only buy things on sale and wouldn't pay his share of items that he thought were luxuries, but he certainly wouldn't have any problem using them or consuming them.

It's funny now, but my Stop and Ask moment was when I found myself hiding toilet paper from him that was better than the generic that he would insist we buy. I said to myself, "What the hell is going on here? Is my life that much out of control that I am hiding toilet paper from my boyfriend?" And then I realized not only did I not love him, I didn't even like him. And more importantly, when I looked in the self-honesty mirror, I didn't like who I was when I was with him. Tim was a symptom of my run-down self-image and self-worth.

Lisa admitted that she had fallen into the role of the "crazy, screwed-up friend" in her friend group.

It was at this point that two people Reached Out to help Lisa. Charles worked with Lisa and adored her as the zany little sister he never had. Lisa and Charles were walking through the city one day when he pointed to the top of a hotel. He said, "Lisa, you are one of my favorite people in the world, but you deserve a lot better caliber of boyfriend than you have been dating. In fact, until you meet a guy who stands on top of that rooftop"—pointing twenty-two stories up—"and proclaims how lucky he is to have you, you shouldn't settle." Lisa was grateful to have such a loving friend—his words gave her the push she needed. She began using the curiosity mindset to brainstorm how she could meet better men.

In fact, Lisa didn't have to look far. She remembered that the husband of her friend Paula had mentioned Erik, a coworker of his who he thought would be a good match for Lisa. Lisa was now aware that her past choices had been wrong, and perhaps her friends had a better sense of what, and who, she deserved. Lisa asked Paula to set up a double-date dinner so she could meet Erik. Before the dinner began, Erik asked to sit on the left side of Lisa because he was left-handed and didn't want to keep nudging her. A small consideration that echoed in Lisa's head.

After the dinner, they arranged another date, which went great. A few days later, Lisa was talking to Erik on the phone when she mentioned that her windshield wipers were not working because of a blown fuse. Within an hour, Erik was at Lisa's boutique, replacing the fuse and the windshield wipers in the middle of a rain shower. One of Lisa's regular customers was watching and said, "I think your knight in shining armor has finally arrived."

After a series of bad relationships, Lisa used the mindset of self-honesty to assess her current situation, and she used curiosity to ask what kind of person she saw herself as and what caliber of man she deserved. She was grateful for the friends in her life who knew she deserved to be with someone who adored her. In the end, Lisa chose to treat herself better and allow a good guy into her life. Fourteen months later, she married Erik, and they are now the parents of two beautiful girls.

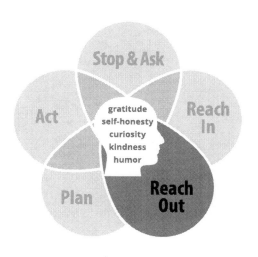

CHAPTER SIX
REACH OUT

—

*A little boy was having difficulty lifting a heavy stone. His father
came along just then. Noting the boy's failure, he asked,
"Are you using all your strength?"
"Yes, I am," the little boy said impatiently.
"No, you are not," the father answered. "I am right here just
waiting, and you haven't asked me to help you."*

—AUTHOR UNKNOWN

Reach Out is what sets apart the *What Matters?!* framework. It's
what makes *What Matters?!* the non-self-help of self-help approaches.
Why? By its very definition, Reach Out cannot be done on your
own. True, at the end of the day you are the one responsible for
your own well-being, but we all need help along the way. Life is

better for you and everyone else when you dare to ask for and offer help. Humans were meant to live in a community, and Reach Out leverages our greatest asset: what we have in common is greater than what divides us.

The Reach Out practice shows us that we can all learn from and teach each other. Bottom line is, it's the people you choose to bring into your life that will help you, and them, to live *What Matters?!*

Are You a Turtle or an Octopus?

Indulge us for a moment as we offer you two symbols that best illustrate Reach Out. Picture a cartoon characterization of a turtle and an octopus (by the way, we are using cartoons because real life images can be a little creepy!). First, focus on the turtle. What do turtles do when they are being attacked? They withdraw into their shells. Think about what happens when you are faced with a stressful situation. Are you a turtle? Now, envision the octopus with its many outstretched tentacles, leveraging all of the resources at its disposal—the exact opposite of a turtle. Reach Out is pretty simple: be an octopus, not a turtle!

Ask yourself, Who can you call in a crisis? If no one comes to mind, we invite you to start flexing your Reach Out muscles.

Our hope is that you will build a network of positive people in your life, people who believe in you and want the best for you. For introverts, Reaching Out is particularly difficult, so even finding one or two go-to folks is a good start.

Beyond your personal connections, there are many professionals who are more than willing to help. Feeling stuck? Why not get a coach? Anxious or depressed? Find a therapist who has the right personality and approach for you. Want a stronger connection to spirit? Try talking to a member of the clergy. The idea is to create a support network that works for you and will help you succeed. Surround yourself with people who can help you live your best life.

REACH OUT: WHAT GETS IN THE WAY?

Our society has embraced the philosophy that asking for help is a sign of weakness. Recent research by Professor Wayne Baker has shown that self-reliance is one of the ten core American values.[44] In short, we have been conditioned to go it alone.

We especially see this dynamic in the workplace. When we coach businesses and other organizations, team members say they're exhausted, isolated, and burned out, in large part because they don't ask one another for help.

Perhaps our obsession with independence started in 1928 when a presidential candidate named Herbert Hoover gave a campaign speech in which he said America was founded on "rugged individualism" and "self-reliance." We have all been raised to admire these qualities, so we go through life trying to fend for ourselves.

In addition to our culture, we face other obstacles in asking for help. Many people hesitate to Reach Out because they're concerned they will need to reciprocate or somehow "owe" the person who has helped them. Others are held back because they worry about imposing—they don't want to "be a bother." As we mentioned earlier in the kindness mindset, the irony is that when others ask us for help, we are not only happy to help, but we also feel a real sense of satisfaction in being able to help others.

Then there are those who believe that "private matters should be kept private." Don't get us wrong. We are not advocating that you shout from the rooftops the most intimate details of your life. However, in the name of so-called propriety, people often suffer in silence. They keep secrets that eat away at them. There is a difference between secrecy and privacy. Remember Karen from a previous chapter? Initially, she felt it was inappropriate to discuss her marital issues with anyone other than her husband—that Reaching Out would be disloyal in some way. The fact is, we all need to vent and unload. External sounding boards are valuable and vital. Be thoughtful about who you confide in, but do not carry your burdens alone. You owe it to yourself, and to your well-being, to share your troubles with a trusted friend, family member, or professional.

THE PROOF IS THERE

There is unequivocal evidence that the quantity and quality of a person's social connections, friendships, relationships with family members, and closeness to neighbors is so intricately related to well-being and personal happiness that they're practically one and the same.[45]

And for all you business leaders, we call on you to actively build Reaching Out into your environment. Not only is it good for individual well-being, it's also good for the bottom line. Indiana University's Philip Podsakoff found that the frequency with which employees help one another predicts sales revenues in pharmaceutical units and retail stores; profits, costs, and customer service in banks; creativity in consulting and engineering firms; productivity in paper mills; and revenues, operating efficiency, customer satisfaction, and performance quality in restaurants.[46]

Getting Started

Okay, now that we've shown the value of Reaching Out, let's talk about some resources that will help you.

Know Your Strengths, Know Your Challenges

When considering where to Reach Out, we encourage you to capitalize on your natural abilities and ask for help with the areas you find difficult. An entrepreneur friend of ours was lamenting the fact that he did not have a good grasp of bookkeeping. We pointed out to him that his gift was thinking of and starting businesses, something that many people wish they could do. He was better off focusing on doing what he did best and hiring a competent bookkeeper to handle the finances. As we like to say, "You can teach a turkey to climb a tree, but you are better off hiring a squirrel."

The Reach Out Toolkit

The Reach Out Toolkit is a simple way to keep you connected to the supportive people in your life. It was created by David for Paul's fortieth birthday, during an especially stressful time in Paul's life. David knew that Paul often did things for himself when, in fact, it would be better for him to Reach Out. So, David wanted to give him a gift that was pragmatic as well as sentimental. Drawing from the abundance of wonderful people in Paul's life, David engraved a Pewter box with the words "Paulie's Toolkit for Living." Inside were multi-colored pieces of paper with a name printed on each one. The names were all the people in Paul's life who loved him, including several who had passed away but were still important sources of strength for him.

When Paul opened the gift, David told him that during challenging times, all he had to do was pull out a name and either call that person or think about how that person believed in him.

CREATING YOUR REACH OUT TOOLKIT

We encourage you to create your own Reach Out Toolkit. Think about the people in your life you can count on for support when you need to achieve a goal, overcome an obstacle, or wade through difficult emotions. You can keep a mental toolkit, but we suggest that you create a physical one. In times of need, our minds often come up short or draw a blank. Your toolkit could be a list on the fridge, or pieces of paper in an envelope or in a small box (small gift box or shoebox).

Here's a sample list of situations that we provide in our workshops to get participants' creative juices flowing about building their toolkit.

WHO CAN YOU CALL . . .

- when feeling a little down and need a pick-me-up?
- to grab something for you at the store?
- for career advice?
- to give you a ride to the airport?
- for financial advice?
- to help you when you are grieving?
- when you need to borrow a thousand dollars?
- when you need a kidney?
- if you are feeling suicidal?
- who will never judge you?
- who believes in you?
- when you need *anything*?

Want to build an actual Reach Out Toolkit? The following exercise will show you how.

REACH OUT TOOKIT

1. Brainstorm a list of situations in which may find yourself where you could benefit from outside assistance.

2. For each situation, identify the person, persons, or group that you could turn to for help. Write a list of these names.

3. Identify any additional people or groups in your life who provide you a sense of support, strength, courage, wisdom, and connections. Add these names to your list.

4. Add to and edit the list over time. The point again is to have the list ready to go, just like you have a physical handyman's tool kit so that when you need a hammer, screwdriver, or wrench it is at the ready.

5. To build a physical toolkit, transcribe the name of each person on your list onto a small slip of paper and place them into a small box (e.g., jewelry box, shoe box).

6. To develop your Reach Out muscles, you may want to randomly pull a name from the toolkit every day and make a quick "hello" phone call to that person.

Have fun with it! If you use an actual box for your toolkit, you can put objects in it that remind you of certain people or that inspire you in some way, like your grandmother's necklace, a slip of paper with the name of an inspirational song, or your lucky penny. Remember to include a wide variety of names or influences in your box; like any other toolkit, you need different tools for different jobs. Think of a tool as anything that gets a job done. In our workshops, we start off everyone's toolkit with a miniature buoy. Why, do you ask? Read on!

Weights and Buoys

Ever notice that some people lift you up while others drag you down? Just like a buoy, positive energy lifts us up—it helps us keep our head above water when life gets choppy. People who bring positive opinions and energy into your life are your buoys. And just like a big, heavy stone, negative energy drags us down, preventing us from moving forward. The people who bring negative opinions and energy into your life are your weights. Notice we say *weights* and not *anchors*, because an anchor serves the purpose of securing a boat; weights, on the other hand, serve no such purpose.

In considering the weights and buoys in your life, it's important to be honest. It's easy to fool yourself when it comes to separating the forces that help you from the forces that hinder you. Sometimes, for example, you might allow the negative people to stick around because you're used to them or because you think it's too hard to break away. You might even make excuses for their behavior instead of holding them accountable.

Your Weights

The thing about weights is, we are allowing them to be weights in our lives. We have two choices: we can either Reach

Out and remove them, or we can Reach In and change how we react to them.

Though we always have a choice about who and what we allow into our lives, sometimes we feel we do not have a choice—think of judgmental in-laws, rebellious children, demanding siblings. In those cases, we suggest you Reach In and change your reaction. Here's an example:

Marsha adored her father-in-law, Alfred, who treated her like a daughter and was a wonderful grandfather to her children. She only had difficulty with him when he pressed his political beliefs, which were the polar opposite of Marsha's and her husband's. It didn't take much for Alfred to set her off, so she had repeatedly asked him to stop discussing politics with her. Inevitably, though, he would say something and her blood pressure would start to rise. Her husband had an easier time not taking the bait. Finally, Marsha accepted that her father-in-law was not going to change; her only alternative, then, was to not react to his comments. She came up with the perfect coping mechanism to distance herself whenever he began talking politics: she would start playing a certain song in her head. Her song of choice was "Crazy" by Patsy Cline.

Consider the following activity to help you let go of the weights in your life.

JETTISONING YOUR WEIGHTS

1. Identify what is weighing you down. It could be a person, thought, behavior, situation, emotion, place, habit—anything that is getting in the way of your living *What Matters?!*

2. Using an indelible marker, write the name of the "weight" on a rock.

3. Find a body of water (e.g., ocean, lake, pond) and toss the rock into its depth. As you release the rock, say the following aloud: "I am no longer allowing _____ (fill in the blank) to weigh me down and interfere with my living *What Matters?!*"

4. In the spirit of Reach Out, many participants in our *What Matters?!* workshops choose to have others witness this symbolic unloading. Some people find that sharing the experience strengthens its impact and fosters accountability.

FRIENDSHIP DIVORCE

The following story is about Maria and how she handled a friendship that was toxic. Here it is in her own words.

I met Mark in the winter of 1997 through a group of mutual friends. He was a charismatic man who was the life of the party. He always said exactly what he was thinking—a characteristic I admired. I have always been concerned about appearances, so I was attracted to his directness and his lack of concern about what others thought of him. Fourteen years my senior, he marched to his own drummer and encouraged me to do the same. We became fast friends, and over the course of fifteen years, he became like family.

Toward the end of our friendship, I began to notice a pattern in our relationship. It seemed that whenever we were together, the bulk of our conversation was him talking about other people. "Can you believe how much so-and-so drinks?" "So-and-so never lifts a finger at a dinner party." "So-and-so can't hold down a job." Although I did my best not to join in, I was as much an accomplice in the negativity as he was by not asking him to stop. Instead, I would just sit there and nod.

I became more and more uncomfortable with our interactions. One of my core values has always been respect. I was being such a hypocrite! Listening to his rants about our mutual friends was a far cry from respectful. I did not like who I was when I was around him, so I began to distance myself as I reevaluated our friendship. Then one day, it got back to me that Mark was talking badly about my husband. Reaching In, I asked myself what I should do. I had a choice: either work with Mark to fix what was broken or leave the relationship. Having a trash-talking friend was no longer acceptable. Mark had become a weight in my life, distracting me from living What Matters?! It was time for a friendship divorce.

I mustered my confidence and went to his house. I sat down and said, "I want to have an important conversation with you that is not easy for me and will likely not be easy for you." I then told him of my unilateral decision to end our friendship, with an explanation as to why. To his credit, Mark owned up to his gossipy behavior and said he was working on it. He also admitted that he, too, was feeling a strain in our relationship. After a lengthy and candid conversation, we hugged each other, wished each other well, and ended our friendship.

What do you think about how Maria navigated her situation? How would you have handled it?

The way we see it, she had three options to enhance her well-being. One, she could have Reached In and changed how she was allowing the relationship to harm her. In other words, she could have continued the friendship and accepted that that was how Mark was wired. Two, she could have tried improving the friendship by giving Mark feedback, which would have required Mark to be open to the discussion and willing to change. Or the third option—the one she chose—she could jettison the weight that the friendship had become. For her, the damage was irreparable and she needed to move on in order to live *What Matters?!*

OTHERS PEOPLE'S DRAMA

Speaking of weights, who among us hasn't been a casualty of getting sucked into others' drama? Your key to well-being? Don't engage! Simply nod politely and keep your mouth shut!

A few years back we discovered this Polish proverb that has become part of our lexicon: "Every time you feel yourself pulled into other people's nonsense, repeat to yourself—Not my circus, not my monkeys." We invite you to make it a part of your What Matters?! toolkit.

YOUR BUOYS

We've dealt with the negative. Now here's the positive. If you want to live *What Matters?!*, you need to surround yourself with positive, supportive people—people who believe in you and your dreams. These "buoys" should be an integral part of your Reach Out Toolkit.

One of David's best friends is Megan, whom he met in college. Megan is David's go-to buoy who he calls when in need of an emotional boost. It doesn't matter if she's talking about renovating her home, playing with her sons, or hanging out with her husband, she always presents it with humor. Whether the chat is two minutes or a half hour, David walks away refreshed, a smile on his face, and chuckling for the rest of the day.

Take a look at the list you wrote for your Reach Out Toolkit. Who is the Megan in your life? Who are additional buoys you'd like to add?

REACH OUT RECESS

One of our favorite tools is Reach Out Recess. Remember recess in elementary school and how much fun it was? Reach Out Recess is when you use your Reach Out Toolkit to contact the important people in your life. By regularly Reaching Out when you are not in need, you are keeping your mental and emotional muscles strong so that you will Reach Out when you are in need. Reaching Out when life is calm also builds a reserve of positive energy that you can draw on when times get rough.

Reach Out Recess is a playful reminder to take the time to Reach Out to the important people in our lives. Who doesn't like getting a call and hearing that someone was thinking of them? You can text or e-mail, but we believe phone calls are the best way to forge a strong emotional connection. The guidelines are simple. If you get voice mail, simply leave a message saying you were thinking of the person. You may want to add that you are practicing Reach Out Recess, a tool you use to stay in touch with the important people in your life, and you can let the person know he or she is one of those important people to you. If you do get the person on the phone, explain that this is a quick call (keep it under five minutes), then quickly explain Reach Out Recess, and lastly, talk about his or her important role in your life. If you haven't spoken in a while, schedule a time to catch up later; Reach Out Recess is meant to be fun and light, not a burden. Otherwise you will never pick up the phone.

CAROL'S STORY: DANCING THROUGH SORROW

Carol was devastated when her husband of more than thirty years died from a heart attack. For the first few months, she was consumed by all the planning and paperwork with the funeral, the well-wishers, and the legal and financial concerns. But when those responsibilities passed, Carol realized she didn't know what came next. Their only son had recently married, and Carol, who had always been independent, had retired, and she and her husband had been looking forward to their next adventure together. Now what?

Although Carol felt like curling up in a ball forever, she stood strong and pondered what she could do with this unexpected new phase in her life. She had no idea what it would entail, but she knew that she needed to take the first step toward healing, so she Reached In and asked herself what would help her move beyond the grief-dance.

Carol had always loved ballroom dancing and had grown up watching her parents, aunts, and uncles dance at family events. For her birthday, Carol's son and daughter-in-law had given her a gift certificate for ballroom dance lessons as a thank you for urging them to take private lessons for their first special dance at their wedding.

Reaching Out, Carol scheduled a lesson, and it turned out to be exactly what she needed: something new, something she had always had a passion for but had never explored. Carol's first lesson led to a series of lessons and a whole lot of fun. She loved the atmosphere and the instructors, who were full of passion and energy. Carol even stepped outside of her comfort zone and signed up for a dance competition, and she placed!

Carol knew that nothing was going to replace her husband or erase her grief. She just needed a way to start moving beyond her pain. And for her, that took the form of the Foxtrot!

THE STAKES CAN BE HIGH

On a serious note, we are personally passionate about Reach Out because of a tragedy that happened to someone dear to us, Jay, who committed suicide in 1998. We can only imagine that asking Jay to "reach out" would have been equivalent to asking a paralyzed person to walk. That's why Reach Out works both ways.

When we are feeling at our best, we must Reach Out to others and let them know that we care and that they are not alone.

If you haven't heard from someone in a while, please pick up the phone. You may find out that there is nothing at all the matter, but you cannot know for certain until you ask. And besides, just letting people know you are thinking about them can build their energy reserve for potential hard times ahead. Remember, it doesn't have to be an hour-long conversation. A thirty-second "just checking in" voice mail will suffice.

ADDITIONAL REACH OUT RESOURCES

Hopefully at this point, you have identified the buoys in your life who are fundamental to your Reach Out practice. We now want to briefly call your attention to some additional Reach Out resources that may be useful for your toolkit.

THE POWER OF GROUPS

Consistent with the Reach Out practice, we encourage you to share your *What Matters?!* journey with another individual—a friend, coworker, or family member. This trusted partner can help you be honest with yourself, offer suggestions, provide encouragement, and foster accountability.

Reach Out goes beyond connecting with individuals. Humans are wired to affiliate, and we benefit greatly from joining groups of like-minded people. Such groups can be organized around common passions, goals, or interests. A wonderful example is our friend Edna, a staple in community theater productions throughout New England. For her, her cast mates are family. Then there's our friend Melissa, who looks forward to teaching her weekly spinning class as a chance to both exercise and connect with the "regulars" during class and at coffee afterward. Our friend Danny is a proud member of a Masonic lodge. Our other friend Jim is part of a group for gay dads.

What's your gig? Volunteer. Join a religious organization. Take a class. Find a local Lean In Circle (www.leanin.org). Remember to be an octopus, not a turtle!

Don't know where to start Reaching Out? Why not try meetup. com, the world's largest network of local groups. Meetup's co-founders, Scott Heiferman and Matt Meeker, wanted to revitalize local communities and help people self-organize. In that vein, Meetup's "About" page says, "People can change their personal world, or the whole world, by organizing themselves into groups that are powerful enough to make a difference."[47]

SUPPORT GROUPS

We also encourage those who are struggling with particular challenges to seek help in the form of support groups. We speak from firsthand experience.

Earlier we referred to Paul's sabbatical in Cape Cod, where the Reach In practice came to life. During that time, Paul also contemplated giving up alcohol for a healthier lifestyle.

Five weeks into the sabbatical, Paul Reached Out to his close friend Billy, a member of Alcoholics Anonymous. For years Paul had considered talking to Billy; now he had finally mustered the courage. Billy's response was compassionate, open, and nonthreatening. He gave Paul a copy of the book *Living Sober*, the ultimate beginner's guide to exploring the nature of alcoholism. Billy also invited him to attend a meeting of Alcoholics Anonymous.

When Paul heard the AA preamble during his first meeting, he knew that he had Reached Out to the right group: "The only requirement for membership is a desire to stop drinking." As of the writing of this book, Paul has not had a drink for over two-and-a-half years and is a proud member of AA.

Though we realize that not everyone can identify with the subject matter of AA, we share this story as an example of the power that reaching out to a group can have. Whether you are coping with bereavement, chronic illness, abuse, weight—whatever the challenge—we encourage you to reach out to a support group.

PETS

If you have pets, consider adding them as an integral part of your Reach Out Toolkit. Is there any being in your life that gives so much and asks so little of you? Cat, dog, bunny, hamster—it doesn't matter. No doubt about it, our furry friends enhance our well-being. Scientific studies show that when you pet an animal, your body releases oxytocin, a neurotransmitter known as the "love drug." Studies also show that pets lower our blood pressure and decrease our heart rates (except during housebreaking!).

FRANCES' STORY

Frances is the thirty-four-year-old granddaughter of Paul's mother's lifelong friend, Marilyn. Although not a blood relative, Frances feels like more of a cousin than a family friend.

In early 2014, Frances Reached Out to us and asked for a loan. She explained that her roommate owed her money and had moved out, leaving her with back rent and unpaid bills. Frances was an extremely self-reliant person, so Reaching Out like this was difficult for her. Since moving out of her grandparents' home at eighteen, Frances had always been a hard worker, holding down multiple jobs. She had never asked for money before. We agreed to give her a loan.

More than a month had passed when Frances called saying that her landlord had evicted her and she didn't know what she was going to do. We became concerned. Frances had a history of drug use and we feared she had relapsed. Rather than give her money, we invited her to come stay with us in Provincetown to regroup for an indefinite period.

Frances, along with Cali, her recently rescued Yorkshire Terrier, arrived at our house in Provincetown on July 9. The date was significant not only because it was Frances' birthday, but also because it was David and Paul's wedding anniversary. That night Frances revealed she was homeless and had spent several nights with Cali, sleeping on a public bench. She blamed herself. Although she was not using, she had surrounded herself with people who were actively using and taking advantage of her good nature.

Sitting in our living room on that July night, we introduced Frances to the What Matters?! framework. Frances realized that she was at a Stop and Ask moment, so she Reached In and committed to a new life.

Outgoing and friendly, Frances began scouring the town for a job, asking everyone she interacted with about potential opportunities. But Provincetown was in full swing at this time of the year and most jobs were already filled. David and Paul's next-door neighbor and dear friend Sue, saw how hard Frances was working and she Reached Out to offer a hand.

Sue was a complete trip for us—she was unlike anyone we had ever met. We felt like we were cooler people just by knowing her. She was a hippie, earth mother, artist, activist, and die-hard nonconformist. She was smart, strong-willed, informed, and passionate about the planet and social justice.

Now with that picture of Sue, imagine her tossing Frances a business card and ordering, "Call this guy, tell him Sue sent you, see if he has anything." The card was that of the captain of Dolphin Fleet, one of Provincetown's famous whale watching cruises. Sue had worked at the Dolphin Fleet for many years.

Frances called the captain, who immediately hired her to work the ships' concession counters. She quickly became a favorite of the tourists and her fellow crew members. As she and Cali walked around the beaches and the town center, she would tell tourists about the cruises and invite them to come visit her on the boat, which many did. Frances's Reaching Out not only benefited her but also the Dolphin Fleet and its guests.

As summer ended, work slowed down. Frances began to wonder what she would do in the off-season—she knew she had to find a more permanent place to live. She had been asking people about rentals, but in the summer, rentals are scarce and expensive. Provincetown, like many resort-based communities, has a shortage of reasonably priced year-round rental housing. Exercising her Reach Out muscles, Frances searched online, talked to coworkers, and responded to ads posted at the supermarket. But given the tremendous demand, everything was snatched up as soon as it was listed.

Frances had no idea that Sue had also been Reaching Out to her network, trying to find a place for her and Cali. Sue had been a local for more than three decades, so her friends knew of housing opportunities before the general public. One particular friend owned a restaurant in town and a few rental properties, which were not glamorous but suitable for year-round living. When this friend could, he gave preference to those in greatest need. Sue told Frances to give him a call about a rental that had just become available. Frances asked David to accompany her to see the cottage. It was a very rustic two-bedroom in the center of town that was both a good price and allowed pets. Frances looked at David and said, "Considering I was homeless several months ago, this place is perfect for me and Cali." Thanks to Sue, Reach Out had once again worked its magic.

Today, Frances continues to thrive in Provincetown. She and Cali are safely nestled in the same humble cottage. Still a favorite on the Dolphin Fleet, Frances has also secured steady employment elsewhere when it's not whale-watching season. She has repaid the loan to David and Paul and purchased a car. She aspires to one day own a home and start a business helping those in need. Sadly, Sue passed away in December 2015. Her legacy of Reach Out lives on in Frances.

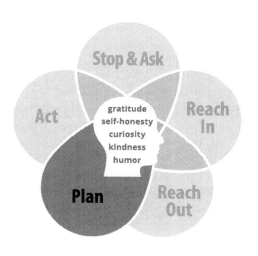

CHAPTER SEVEN
PLAN

What Matters?! is about living a conscious and intentional life where you are thriving more and stressing less. So far we have discussed practices to enhance awareness of how you are living now, and offered you approaches for the current circumstances in your life.

Anticipating the future has almost a gravitational pull, but we have tried to keep the discussion to the present—because it is in this moment that we create the internal circumstances which connect us deeply to ourselves and the people around us. Now, we are ready to turn our attention to consciously and intentionally creating the future. We do this through the Plan practice.

BIG P. VERSUS LITTLE P.

The Plan practice is about envisioning the future that you want to create for yourself and determining how you will create it. It's not about drawing up a business plan or a life plan or a five-year plan or a strategic plan (unless that's what matters to you). The idea of planning can freak some people out; so if you are freaking out right now, relax. Or if you love to plan, great. We invite you to entertain our spin on the concept.

It could be a little P. plan, like deciding what you're going to do five minutes from now, or next week, or next month. If you wake up in the morning and decide you want boneless chicken for dinner rather than say, a Big Mac, you are little P. planning to achieve what matters to your health. When you decide at what time you will go to the grocery store (or the barbeque joint) to pick up your boneless chicken, that's also little P. planning.

A big P. plan might be getting gastric bypass surgery or becoming vegan. Other big P. examples include planning for your next career move, or for retirement, or for an empty nest. Like the rest of *What Matters?!*, Planning is personal. The time horizon that you choose is completely up to you. Whether it's five days from now or five years from now, all we ask is that you choose a direction for your future as well as the potential paths for how you might get there.

CREATING A PLAN

Before we continue with Plan, let's review what we've covered so far. We began with Stopping and Asking what matters to you and how much your daily living reflects what you say is important. Reaching In, you identified some areas you may want to modify. Reaching Out, you gained others' perspectives.

At this point in the *What Matters?!* process, the overachiever in you might come out, and you write a list of *everything* you want to change: ditch the job you hate, lose twenty pounds, cut down on drinking, break up with that friend who is sucking the life out of you, spend less money, go back to school, volunteer more. You feel the excitement in you building. Anything is possible. Look out world! And then BAM—"reality" sets in.

Ditch the job? But I've got a mortgage to pay, kids to send to college, aging parents to care for, retirement to save for. Lose twenty pounds? Who has time to go to the gym? Cut down on drinking? But my social life revolves around cocktail parties. That friend I want to break up with? We've known each other for years and years. Spend less money? I've already cut to the bone. Go back to school? Way too overwhelming. Volunteer more? I'm not passionate about any cause.

Time to slow down, take a deep breath, and Plan. For those of you who like structure, the following worksheet has a framework for planning that uses the entirety of the *What Matters?!* model. For those of you who don't like structure, or are already master planners, we invite you to review this worksheet, anyway. Of course, like the rest of this book, the choice is yours.

PLAN

STEP 1

As your first step in planning, Reach In and identify an area of your life you wish to address. You can do so by asking yourself any or all of the following questions:

- What is something in your life (behavior, person, habit, thought/belief, fear, circumstance) that is no longer working for you?

- What is something that is working for you that you might want to enhance or have more of?

- What do you aspire to? In other words, what is a goal or outcome you wish to accomplish?

If you are having trouble identifying an area that you wish to make a plan, consider Reaching Out and getting some input. No need to agonize, though. You can always go back later and plan for some different areas. Just because you put a plan together doesn't obligate you to implement the plan. In fact, the exercise of planning often brings clarity about other areas that might warrant more focus.

STEP 2

Next, write the specific change.

STEP 3

Envision what your life would be like were this change to be in place or goal achieved. What is happening in your life? What is your level of energy? How would people describe you? What is your level of satisfaction?

STEP 4

Now, identify the obstacles/challenges preventing you from making this change or achieving this goal.

STEP 5

For each obstacle/challenge identify whether it is something that you need to "accept" (things beyond your control, external circumstances) or "change" (things you can do something about, internal circumstances).

STEP 6

For each item that you labeled as "change," identify whether that change is something that is best accomplished by "Reaching In" or "Reaching Out." It could be both.

STEP 7

Identify the Reach In, Reach Out and any other actions that you need to take to create the change or accomplish the goal. Be sure to attach "by when" dates to each action.

STEP 8

Determine how you will hold yourself accountable to taking these actions (see our next chapter for some tips).

STEP 9

Put your plan into action. Monitor your follow-through and course-correct as necessary. (Nervous? You'll love the next chapter!)

HELP, I'M STUCK!

Planning, especially big P. planning, requires envisioning the future. But what, you may ask, do I do if I don't have a vision? In fact, many of our clients come to us because they do not know where they want to go. Like driving on a foggy evening, their vision of what lies ahead is obscured. For many, that is a scary way to go through life, so they try to force clarity. But the more they try to force it, the less they are able to think clearly. Their anxiety of not knowing feeds on itself and creates further mind blocks—a vicious cycle.

In these cases, you may want to answer the following Reach In questions to help create your vision. You may also want to Reach Out and discuss them with someone important to you.

WORKING IT

- ✓ Imagine yourself as a ninety-year-old. You are in excellent health, both physically and mentally, and are content and satisfied. You've been invited to speak to a class of college students about "Living Your Best Life." You are preparing your remarks. What advice do you want to give these young people?
- ✓ You've been given a month to do anything you want, go anywhere you want, be with anyone you want. You're well-rested at the start of the month, having just returned from a vacation. You don't have any chores to do or any obligations, and you have whatever resources you need. How will you spend this month, and why? What is important to you and how is that reflected in your choices?
- ✓ You have the chance to take one period of your life and live it over again, changing your choices, actions, and insights. What period would you choose? What would you do differently, and why?

Still don't have a picture? That's perfectly natural. You can't force the vision. Sometimes the Plan is to simply trust that the vision will unfold, to sit in the presence of the unknown and continue to Stop and Ask. In the discomfort of not knowing, you can use your Reach In and Reach Out tools to manage the anxiety and develop patience and optimism that clarity will emerge. From that calmer, less reactive place, you can then take small steps that will help your vision come to life.

PAY ATTENTION!

The greatest opportunities for living *What Matters?!* often aren't part of your original plan—they present themselves unexpectedly. Stay awake and aware. You never know what the universe is going to bring your way. Russian poet and novelist Boris Pasternak said, "When a great moment knocks on the door of your life, it is often no louder than the beating of your heart, and it is very easy to miss it."[48]

Mimi has spent most of her career as an accomplished writer, but she temporarily stopped writing to care for her aging mother. When she was ready to return to the workforce, she couldn't find a writing job. She'd always had a passion for baking and was very good at it. As it so happens, the Whole Foods near her house was looking for a cake decorator. Mimi applied and is today happily employed doing work she loves. Listen to your strengths and keep your eyes open. You never know where you might find an opportunity that wasn't part of your plan!

DON'T FORGET TO FEEL WHEN YOU PLAN

Most traditional planning focuses on the external circumstances you want to create. For example, in ten years I will have a PhD, be earning $120,000 per year, have relocated to California, and be in a serious relationship. Just as importantly, though, we need to ask ourselves what the internal experience will be once we've achieved our goals. Ask yourself, What will my life feel like once I've reached my destination? For example, in ten years I will eagerly jump out of bed every morning, manage challenges with an adventurous spirit, and enjoy a strong connection to the people in my life.

You can then work backward from this internal goal and decide how you want to feel along the way, because Planning isn't just about the future. A critical part of it is choosing how you want to experience working toward your goals. What are you willing to say "yes" to? What are you willing to say "no" to? What tradeoffs are you willing to make? What are you willing to forgo?

What good is it to attain a goal if, by the time you get there, you have had the life sucked out of you? What Matters?! is about savoring the moment rather than anticipating and trying to control the future. We're not saying you should abandon your goals, but we do want you to ask yourself, What's the use of going after something if I'm going to be miserable along the way? You might get there and be content for a moment, then discover that your contentedness has worn off and you find yourself compulsively pursuing the next goal.

We are not saying don't strive. By all means, strive (if that's what matters to you), but recognize that there are two ways to achieve a goal: you can do it miserably (as an ordeal), or you can do it while savoring each moment of the journey (as an adventure). Setting long-term goals and working hard to achieve them is, in many ways, a given; the variable is if you will allow the journey to feed your soul. This is the difference between "I'll be happy when" versus "I'll be happy while."

We saw this difference painfully illustrated during a workshop we conducted for a group of Harvard undergraduates. While we were discussing the practice of Plan, one of the students, a sophomore, raised her hand.

STUDENT: *I know that I want to be a pediatric neurosurgeon. That's what matters to me. To get there, the next fifteen years of my life are spoken for. I will need to work my butt off. It's going to be a never-ending treadmill.*

DAVID: *Let me ask you something. You're a sophomore now. If the rest of your undergraduate experience was the best that it could possibly be, can you describe what that would look like?*

STUDENT: *Well, I'd do really well in my classes, and I wouldn't be as stressed out as I am now.*

DAVID: *And what would it be like to be less stressed out? What's possible?*

STUDENT: Well, I'd probably enjoy my classes a whole lot more. I'd sleep better, too. I'd also be less preoccupied in general.

DAVID: Anything else?

STUDENT: Well, yes. I'd have more fun with my roommates. They are great people—always trying to get me to go to football tailgates—but I've just got too much work.

DAVID: How important is it for you to enjoy your classes, sleep better, be less preoccupied, and have more fun with your roommates?

STUDENT: I'd like that, but the fact is, I'm a stress monger. It's how I'm wired. It just goes with the territory of being a premed.

DAVID: I get it. You seem resigned to the fact that this needs to be how it is. But let me ask you this. If there were just one thing you could do to reduce your stress level, what would that be?

STUDENT: I really don't know.

DAVID: Come on. Work with me. One thing.

STUDENT: Well, music really soothes me.

DAVID: Great. Any particular kind?

STUDENT: I love old-school jazz and R&B. You know, like Ella Fitzgerald and Ray Charles.

DAVID: *So, music soothes you. How can you bring more music into your life?*

STUDENT: *Well, since I've been having trouble sleeping, what if I listened to some chill-out music before bed?*

DAVID: *What if you did? What would that give you?*

STUDENT: *I might sleep better. Hey, I just had an idea. What if I spent five minutes every morning listening to music before class, too? That might be a calm way to start my day.*

DAVID: *Willing to give it a shot?*

STUDENT: *Absolutely.*

DAVID: *Who can you reach out to encourage this new habit?*

STUDENT: *One of my roommates really likes the same kind of music. I could see if perhaps she would listen with me. Or at the very least, I could ask her to remind me to do it.*

DAVID: *Wonderful. Here's the thing. You've set some ambitious goals with med school, but don't you think you owe it to yourself to make the journey tolerable—and dare I say—enjoyable?*

STUDENT: *With how I'm wired, I just never thought it was possible.*

DAVID: *What do you think now?*

STUDENT: *Well, at least I have some hope. In fact, now I'm motivated to look for other ways to keep myself sane over the next few years.*

DAVID: *And my hope for you is that you'll be more than just sane, that you will actually thrive on your journey to becoming a doctor. You won't get these fifteen years of your life back.*

STUDENT: *Thank you for reminding me of that.*

You don't have to be a college premed to sympathize with that scenario. In what ways are you like this student? How are you abandoning yourself for the sake of achieving a goal? How much of that is acceptable? Where have you crossed a line? What kinds of practices do you need to put into place to ensure that the journey toward your goal is an adventure and not an ordeal? Are you mindfully choosing?

All this is to remind you to add Stop and Ask moments into your plan. How you feel during the journey will determine if the destination was worthwhile. Consider the words of Eckhart Tolle, author of *The Power of Now*:

> *Do you treat this moment as if it were an obstacle to be overcome? Do you feel you have a future moment to get to that is more important? Almost everyone lives like this most of the time. Since the future never arrives, except as the present, it is a dysfunctional way to live. It generates a constant undercurrent of unease, tension, and discontent. It does not honor life, which is Now and never not Now.*[49]

WHOSE MEASURING STICK ARE YOU USING?

In planning for the "not now," we encourage you to Reach Out for input. However, it is important to remember that, as the master of your own destiny, you are in charge of deciding what is best for you. Keep in mind that not all advice has equal weight, and every person's perspective is unique.

Consider, for example, a piece of advice Charles Wheelan gives in his book *10½ Things No Commencement Speaker Has Ever Said*: "Your Parents Don't Want What Is Best for You." He continues, "They want what is good for you, which isn't always the same thing. There is a natural instinct to protect our children from risk and discomfort, and therefore to urge safe choices. Theodore Roosevelt—soldier, explorer, president—once remarked, 'It is hard to fail, but it is worse never to have tried to succeed.' Great quote, but I am willing to bet that Teddy's mother wanted him to be a doctor or a lawyer."[50]

This instinct to protect is not limited to parents. Well-meaning friends, family members, coworkers, and trusted professionals have no shortage of opinions about what is best for us. And what is best to them stems from their own life experiences, beliefs, and social norms—not a bad thing. But if their advice is stressing you out, remember that what they are saying may not be *your* truth. Reach In, get honest with yourself, and choose what is best for you.

Brad was upset after discussing his retirement with a financial advisor who told him he was "behind the eight ball." We should mention that Brad is twenty-four years old, he graduated from a great engineering school, and he started his first job within the past year. Behind the eight ball? Really?

Yes, by all means, plan for retirement or any other part of your life you envision for yourself, but be careful not to overdose on Planning, which can become an obsession that robs you of your life.

Knowing When to Say "Yes" and "No"

What Matters?! is about taking accountability for leading your life. Former British Prime Minister Tony Blair said, "The art of leadership is saying no, not saying yes. It is very easy to say yes."[51] So, in planning for the future, it is important to have clear guidelines for your choices. What will you say "yes" to? What will you say "no" to?

Ezra's Story: You Can't Always Choose Family

Ezra is vice president of Investor Relations at a biotechnology company that recently went public, and one of his responsibilities is to brief the executive team for each quarterly earnings call. One such call was scheduled for a Thursday on the same week when Ezra's son, Sam, would be receiving his Eagle Scout rank at an out-of-state ceremony. Ezra had planned to brief the executive team on Tuesday, then attend Sam's ceremony on Wednesday, and return in time for the quarterly earnings call on Thursday. Though hectic, the schedule would allow Ezra to honor his commitments to work and family.

But on Tuesday morning, Ezra discovered that over half of the executive team had been delayed overseas and was unavailable. The briefing would have to be rescheduled for Wednesday, the same day as Sam's Eagle Scout ceremony. Ezra approached his boss and explained the situation. Even though his boss was empathetic, he could not help. Briefing the team was critical to the success of the entire company, and Ezra was the only person qualified to do it.

Ezra was sick to his stomach. Sam's ceremony was a once-in-a-lifetime moment—only five percent of all Boy Scouts achieve Eagle Scout! Ezra would feel awful if he missed it, but what could he do?

Reaching In, Ezra and his wife considered the options. Their conclusion? He'd have to disappoint Sam. For them, the financial well-being of their family (i.e., job security) trumped attending a family member's milestone. A difficult choice for all, but one guided by a specific plan. Months before, Ezra and his wife had completed the What Matters?! *planning tool below.*

EZRA'S "YES'S" AND "NO'S"

I SAY "YES" TO...	I SAY "NO" TO...
• Family dinners ten nights per month	• Earning less than $150,000 as a household per year
• Dad traveling for work 50 percent of the time	• Mom working outside the home
• After-school jobs for the kids	• Cell phones at meals
• Attending church as a family at least two times per month	• Dad jeopardizing his health
• Biking as a family two times per month	• Blame and negativity in our home
• The kids sharing a bedroom	• Television at meals
• Ensuring laughter in our home	• Potato chips, soda, and high-sugar foods in the house
• Respecting one another	• Having secrets
• Sharing our feelings	• Raising our voices

Now, if you'd like, it's your turn to decide on your yes's and no's.

Yes's and No's

In the chart below, indicate what you need to say "yes" to and what you need to say "no" to in order to guide you in making choices to live *What Matters?!*

I SAY "YES" TO...	I SAY "NO" TO...

Some Helpful Planning Tips

Even though your plan is unique to you, here are some suggestions to consider:

- Track your progress. Identify milestones along the way that will tell you whether you are going in the right direction. (These aren't just about whether you have achieved a tangible outcome, but whether the journey itself is allowing you to live what matters.)
- Don't hold yourself hostage to the plan. Course-correct as needed.
- Allow for things to unfold organically. You never know what the universe is going to bring your way.
- Remember to celebrate small wins.
- Push outside of your comfort zone! --
- Set aside at least five minutes every day for planning. (This is different from the time you have set aside to Stop and Ask and Reach In.)
- Make a daily prioritized To Do list.
- Set weekly, monthly, yearly goals.
- Schedule vacations.
- Decide what you will say "yes" to.
- Decide what you will say "no" to.
- Create a financial plan.
- Schedule downtime, fun time, and leisure time.
- Determine a set time every day after which you will no longer check e-mail or conduct business.
- Identify and eliminate your time wasters.

PEGGY'S STORY: PLANNING IN INCREMENTS

Peggy, a single young woman in her twenties, was set to graduate at the top of her class in nursing school. As she contemplated her future, she met with her faculty advisor to explore her options. In their first meeting, the professor asked, "So, where do you see yourself in five years?" Five years? Peggy couldn't even fathom the next five months! He encouraged her to contemplate the question and scheduled another meeting for a couple of weeks later.

The next session arrived, but Peggy still had nothing. Same with the session after that. Try as she might, Peggy could not envision her future beyond the next few months. While she liked studying nursing, how could she foresee that she'd want to stay in the field? Who knew where she would be living? Would she be in a relationship? Would she even want to be in one?

The more Peggy sat with the "five year question," the more anxious she became. Her advisor grew frustrated. Peggy had incredible potential; she could be a powerhouse in the field. He interpreted her lack of clarity as lack of commitment and told her that there was nothing more he could do.

Peggy interviewed for a series of jobs, but she left each one feeling more and more anxious. Like her advisor, they all wanted to know her career aspirations. The only thing she knew is that she wanted to give nursing a try. She felt nauseous at the thought of accepting any of the job offers.

Just when Peggy thought there was no hope, she came across an organization that hired traveling nurses for three-month temporary assignments. Finally, something that resonated with her. Not only could she give nursing a try, but she could experiment living in a new place.

After graduating, Peggy took a three-month assignment in Nashville, Tennessee. To her delight, she discovered that she did enjoy hands-on nursing. Nashville was a pretty nice place, too! As the end of the assignment neared, Peggy contemplated her next move. She liked it there and was offered another three-month assignment. Before she knew it, she had extended two more times and a year had past.

The hospital was thrilled with her work and offered her a full-time job. Management painted a picture for her of a flourishing career at their facility. Familiar feelings of anxiety returned. Again Peggy felt paralyzed thinking about her future in anything more than three-month increments. Much to the hospital's disappointment, she declined the full-time offer. She did, however, sign up for another three-month rotation.

As the end of that rotation neared, the traveling nurse agency that employed Peggy presented her with an opportunity for a three-month assignment in San Francisco. "Well," she thought, "I'm enjoying nursing, and San Francisco sounds great, so why not?" Off she went, reupping for four rotations as she had in Nashville. Déjà vu. Delighted with her performance, the San Francisco hospital asked her to come aboard full-time and promised an exciting career ahead. Once again, Peggy declined. While she had grown reasonably sure over the past two years that nursing was her life's work, she still couldn't contemplate planning in more than three-month increments.

Ten years later, Peggy continues to thrive as a traveling nurse. She has worked in more than ten states, working in three-month increments. She has developed a network of friends throughout the country and maintains deep ties with her family. In addition, her flexible schedule has afforded her the opportunity to participate in annual month-long service trips to underdeveloped countries. "While it's certainly not for everyone, planning my life in three-month increments works for me. That could very well change if I were ever to have children. However, I trust that all will unfold as it is supposed to. I just need to pay attention to what feels true for me." Peggy plans her own way. You get to plan your own way.

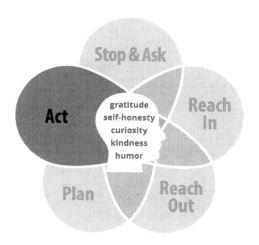

CHAPTER EIGHT
ACT

After you have Stopped and Asked, Reached In and Reached Out, and Planned, now you need to Act. For some people, this is the scariest of the five practices—but it doesn't have to be.

Entrepreneural coach Donna Netwig introduced us to the philosophy of imperfect action, which we love. Imperfect action is about taking a step forward without everything being perfectly aligned. The idea is to act on something, knowing that it is not flawless but that you can adjust as you move forward.

Holding back in the name of "getting it right" does not serve you. Sure, you may fail. But wouldn't you rather risk failure than not pursue what matters to you?

Are you a perfectionist? If so, how does your need for perfection get in the way of your own well-being? How does it impact others? Not only can your actions be imperfect, they can be small actions, too. The important thing is that you intentionally choose to do something and then you do it. Use what you learn from that experience to inform what you do next. After a while, you'll come closer and closer to hitting the bull's-eye. Professional hockey player Wayne Gretzky said, "You miss 100 percent of the shots you don't take." The practice of Act encourages you to take your best shot at living *What Matters?!* Because no one else can do it for you.

One of the things that we hope you have gotten from the *What Matters?!* framework is that living consciously and intentionally is the key to well-being. Nowhere is this more applicable than in choosing what actions you will take, or—just as importantly—knowing what actions you will *not* take. In a sense, the four practices leading up to Act are also forms of action. Taken collectively, they raise your awareness about how you are living, so you can thrive in your current circumstances and envision your best future. Act is all that and more. It is what moves us from envisioning to doing so that we can bring our mindful choices to life.

Big A. Action versus Little A. Action

As with the other practices, we want to call your attention to *little* and *big*. Little A. "a" actions are those that help you to thrive within your current circumstances. For example, perhaps you are someone who tends to isolate and you've committed to calling someone every day for a five-minute Reach Out Recess. That is little A. action. Other examples of little A. action include swapping your morning blueberry muffin for some fruit and yogurt, being curious rather than upset about a conflict at work, and turning off the television to play a game with your family.

Then there are big A. actions, those that propel you forward and transform your future. Tired of being isolated, you join an online dating site. (Your Mr. or Mrs. Right could be one click away!) You step up at work and have that difficult conversation with your boss. You put your house on the market, or you go on a long-overdue vacation without your laptop. If you are taking a gulp right now, that's perfectly normal. Big A. actions tend to push us out of our comfort zones.

Think about your own situation. What's a little A. action you can do within the next twenty-four hours that will help you live *What Matters?!* How about a big A. action that you can take in the next month? Go ahead and write them down below. We dare you!

WORKING IT

My little A. action in the next twenty-four hours:

_____

My big A. action in the next month:

_____

ACTION VERSUS MOTION: A CAVEAT

Never mistake activity for achievement.

—JOHN WOODEN, BASKETBALL PLAYER AND COACH

Earlier in the book we talked about how being busy has become a badge of honor. As we invite you now to take action, some of you may be tempted to bite off more than you can chew. And if lots of action is what matters to you—in other words, if it enhances your well-being—have at it! However, when action is taken to an extreme, it can also undermine well-being by seducing us into living as "human doings" rather than human beings. Only you know the optimal volume and pace of action that reflects what matters to you. Use the self-honesty mindset and choose intentionally.

We also want to distinguish between being in motion and taking action. When you are living in motion rather than taking intentional action, you will probably wake up one day and realize that your life has been living you instead of you living it—that you have been on autopilot and squandered time you can never get back. Action, on the other hand, is about conscious and intentional choice about where you want to spend the valuable currency of your life. Budget wisely!

What Gets in the Way of Action
Getting It "Right" Is Often "Getting Stuck"

Many impediments to moving forward first appear as rational excuses. "I can't join the dating site because I don't have a good profile picture." "I can't take the Zumba class because I have no rhythm." "I can't apply for that manager job because I've never managed before." We invite you to take a moment and Reach In. Where might you be living in analysis paralysis?

The following coaching dialogue is quite typical of those holding themselves back from action. Before reading the conversation, think of a situation in your life where you are delaying moving forward and how Jim's predicament may mirror your own.

JIM: *I really need to get going on my job search, but I'm feeling stuck.*

PAUL: What's going on?

JIM: *I just can't get my résumé right.*

PAUL: Right? What do you mean?

JIM: *I need to figure out a way to position the gap in my experience—it looks bad.*

PAUL: Why not just tell it how it is?

JIM: No one will look at me.

PAUL: You seem really sure of that.

JIM: *That's the way of the world.*

PAUL: *Jim, let me ask you something. What is the consequence of not finishing your résumé?*

JIM: Well, without it I can't apply for jobs.

PAUL: How are you planning on sourcing potential opportunities?

JIM: Primarily through networking.

PAUL: How much networking are you doing now?

JIM: *None.*

PAUL: *Why is that?*

JIM: *Because I don't have an up-to-date résumé.*

PAUL: *Let me get this straight. The way you plan to find a job is through networking, but you won't let yourself network until your résumé is finished. Tell me why you are choosing this route.*

JIM: *Well, I'm likely to have better success networking with a stronger résumé. You only get one turn at bat, you know.*

PAUL: *So, until your résumé is buttoned up, networking is out of the question.*

JIM: *"Out of the question" is a little strong.*

PAUL: *Okay, where are some possible places you could network immediately, even without a résumé?*

JIM: *Well, my old fraternity brother is doing some exciting stuff in cloud computing that really interests me. I suppose I could reach out to him and grab lunch.*

PAUL: *Even without a résumé?*

JIM: *Sure, he's my buddy.*

PAUL: *Anyone else fall into this camp of people you can contact before your résumé is complete?*

JIM: *Well, my sister-in-law's sister is with a headhunting firm. I suppose I could reach out to her—hey, she might even be able to give me some advice on my résumé.*

PAUL: *Great. When will you contact your fraternity brother and your sister-in-law's sister?*

JIM: *I could do that today. In fact, I will.*

PAUL: *Good for you. Just for kicks, why don't you e-mail me after you've reached out to them and let me know how it went.*

JIM: *Will do.*

PAUL: *And, Jim, one more thing. I see that you are putting a lot of credence in your résumé. I'm not saying that you are wrong, but it's holding you back. May I make a suggestion?*

JIM: *Sure. You've already got me contacting two people I wasn't ready to before this conversation. Who knows what I might get out of your next suggestion!*

PAUL: *Set a deadline for finishing your résumé. Call it Version One if you like, but finish the damn thing and start using it. The gap is always going to be the gap. Unless you are blindly applying for jobs on websites where a program is searching for gaps, your résumé isn't going to disqualify you. Your résumé doesn't get you a job, you and your network do.*

JIM: *Thanks for the reality check. I really appreciate it.*

PROCRASTINATION

Procrastination is when we know what it is we need to do and we have the wherewithal to do it, but we keep putting it off. For big A. actions, procrastination often comes from fear. Perhaps you are putting off that important conversation with your friend, family member, or colleague because you don't like conflict.

For little A. stuff, procrastination is often caused by lack of motivation. Doing laundry, cleaning out the garage, grocery shopping . . . usually the nonsexy things that aren't satisfying but are necessary to keep life on track.

Believe it or not, research shows that procrastination impairs your health. A study in *Psychology Today* found that college students who procrastinated caught more colds and flu, had more gastrointestinal problems, and suffered from insomnia.[52] Who knew a pile of laundry could wreak such havoc!

While there is no magic solution for procrastination, you may want to try some of these suggestions:

- Reach out to a friend, family member, or colleague and explain where in your life you are procrastinating. Tell them that if you don't complete what you are avoiding by a certain date, you will donate one hundred dollars* to the charity of their choice. (*Whatever the amount, it should feel consequential to you.)
- For larger tasks, break them into smaller pieces and do them a little at a time.
- Envision what you are going to feel like once you have done what you've been putting off.
- Identify a reward that you can give yourself once you have taken the action you have been procrastinating. Buy yourself

an ice cream, go to a movie, purchase those shoes you've had your eye on. The reward should be proportionate to the magnitude of the action you've been avoiding. (No flying to Hawaii for having cleaned out the garage!)

WORKING IT

What's something you've been procrastinating that is getting in the way of living *What Matters?!* It could be a big A. or a little A. What's it costing you? When will you do it? Really, we mean it, when will you?

If you are having a hard time tackling the less glamorous stuff, a little gratitude can help get you going. Paul had a family friend, Toby, who was confined to a wheelchair—the result of polio. She was truly one of the most upbeat people. One day, Paul came home from school to find his mother on her hands and knees, happily humming to herself as she scrubbed the bathroom floor. When he asked her how on earth she could be so pleasant doing such a gross task, she said, "Honey, what my Toby wouldn't do to be able to scrub her own floors. And although it's not my favorite thing, I'm choosing to do this. It's part of being your mother." Is it any wonder that we've dedicated this book to her?

FEAR OF FAILURE

Of course, what may be holding you back from Acting is not only the drudgery of a task but also the fear of failure. Fear of failure is natural—after all, everyone fears failure a little—but when we start fearing it a lot, we lose our ability to Act.

The other day a friend of ours posted a quote on Facebook from Jon Sinclair: "Failure is a bruise, not a tattoo." That sentence got us to thinking about how different people relate to failure. Does it devastate you and hold you back from taking more action? Or do you see it as an energizing opportunity to learn, course-correct, and move forward?

CLAIRE AND TOM'S STORY: CRAFTING THEIR OWN DEFINITION OF SUCCESS

Tom was a landscape designer at Thompson's Nursery. He and his wife Claire had three young children and dreamed of running their own business. Thompson's Nursery was a major retailer of Christmas trees and started selling them the weekend after Thanksgiving. Claire had an idea of how to capitalize on the captive audience of tree buyers who would also be in need of gifts. With Mr. Thompson's permission, she opened up a boutique in one of the nursery's empty buildings and sold holiday gifts as well as offered a large selection of ribbons and elaborate bows she had made to adorn the gift boxes for a modest additional charge.

After the first busy weekend, Tom, exhausted from selling trees, went to see how many gifts Claire had sold. Claire informed him that she didn't sell many of the gifts. Obviously disappointed for his wife, he tried to console her. To his surprise, Claire was not upset at all. She said, "I said we didn't sell many gifts, but so many people were interested in the beautiful ribbons and bows that I sold all of them." She looked at her husband and declared, "We are out of the gift business and in the ribbons and bows business!" Rather than dwelling on her failure to sell gifts, Claire instead saw it as a chance to course-correct and continue moving forward.

Selling ribbons and bows led to selling craft supplies, until they took over the entire Thompson Nursery and then relocated to a *larger property. Together Claire and Tom built one of the largest independent craft businesses in Massachusetts—they were pioneers in what is now a $30 billion industry.*

What is your reaction to Claire and Tom's story? Did they fail? At Paul's twenty-fifth college reunion, Oprah Winfrey gave a commencement speech and said, "Failure is just life trying to move us in another direction."

TRUST YOUR INTUITION

Intuition is defined as what one knows or considers likely out of an instinctive feeling rather than conscious reasoning.[53] In other words, we don't have to analyze everything; sometimes we can listen to urges. Whether it's creating the first wheel or building the first rocket to Mars, every invention known to humankind has required a good dose of intuition. Even the Ziploc bag!

As Albert Einstein said, "The intuitive mind is a sacred gift and the rational mind is a faithful servant. We have created a society that honors the servant and has forgotten the gift."

WORKING IT

Can you think of a time when you didn't follow your intuition and you later wished you had? What kept you from doing so?

ARE YOU ACTING OR REACTING?

In addition to paying attention to how things fall into place and trusting your intuition, how else can you determine whether your proposed action will best serve you? Here's where it helps to ask yourself about the underlying motive for taking (or not taking) the action you are considering.

In general, we believe that action (or inaction) motivated by fear and anxiety is detrimental to long-term well-being.

Don't get us wrong. If your house is on fire or a tidal wave is approaching, run to the nearest exit! However, we remind you of the saber-toothed tigers we mentioned earlier in the book. Make sure you are acting (or not acting) for reasons that will help you create your best life. Fear-based decisions may alleviate your anxiety in the short-term, but they tend to carry with them negative long-term consequences.

SONYA'S STORY: A FEAR-BASED DECISION AND ITS CONSEQUENCES

After ten years on the job, Sonya, a forty-year-old single woman, was laid off as an editor at a global business publication. She was given six-months severance. Three months into her unemployment, she was offered work at a fashion magazine. The position paid 15 percent more than her previous job, and her commute would be an easy twenty minutes.

One of the things Sonya had enjoyed about her previous position was the intellectual stimulation of editing business articles. She also liked working as part of a team. While the new opportunity would engage her editing skills, the content of the work held no great appeal to her, and she'd be working on her own.

The job market in Sonya's field was extremely competitive. So far in her three-month search, she had interviewed with three organizations. None of these had resulted in an offer. She was beginning to get antsy. Her severance would run out in three months and she had no other opportunities on the horizon.

Sonya went to dinner with her friend Nancy to discuss the situation. When Sonya told her about the offer from the fashion magazine, Nancy exclaimed, "How can you even think about not taking it? That's one of the most prominent magazines out there. You really think you are going to find something better in this market? You're a single woman approaching middle age. You need to be realistic."

Sonya replied, "I suppose you are right. Hey, I could even learn to enjoy the fashion industry. I'll never know unless I try. And as for working without a team, I can find other outlets for connecting with people. Not to mention, a 15 percent raise is pretty darn good, especially in this market."

Sonya convinced herself to take the job. She knew deep down that it wasn't a great fit, but the thought of her severance ending in three months in a tight market was clouding her judgment.

A month into the job, Sonya realized she had made a terrible mistake. Working without a team, she felt isolated and unsupported. Her feelings of frustration and resentment against the content of her work intensified with every subsequent assignment. As the months rolled by, she lost more and more *motivation. She was now missing deadlines and submitting low-quality work. Sonya had high standards for herself and was deeply disturbed by her job performance. But try as she might, she could not get out of her rut. Anxiety and sleepless nights became her norm.*

Completely beaten down, Sonya was fired after eight months on the job. It would take her four months and extensive coaching to recover from the ordeal. After reflecting on her experience, she knew that she had taken the job out of fear and peer pressure. Her intuition had told her that it wasn't the right fit, but the desperate voice of scarcity had been louder. Having learned the hard way, she vowed never again to let fear dictate her life decisions.

Sonya is now happily employed editing articles at a political publication. She is part of a great team and looks forward to going to work every day.

Flowing vs. Forcing

How do you decide that the action you are taking isn't the best action after all? In other words, when does applying effort become forcing something that wasn't meant to be as opposed to flowing with reality? Knowing when to stop taking action is a subtle but important skill.

We call these "IKEA moments," named after the Swedish furniture store. IKEA furniture is assembled by the purchaser, as many people know all too well. Each piece of furniture comes with an instruction pamphlet as well as parts to assemble. Sometimes the process goes smoothly and the piece comes together easily, but other times (perhaps too frequently), you miss a step or use the wrong screw or lose a peg. At times like this, it's best to take a break, or at the very least to take a deep breath, accept that you may have gone about it the wrong way, then take a closer look at the instructions, course-correct, and finish assembling. The alternative is to become frustrated and force the parts together, which could cause irreparable damage and the piece never looks exactly right.

While we realize that handling life is much more important than assembling furniture, we invite you to reflect metaphorically on the IKEA moments you've experienced.

Working It

1. Where have you tried to force something to happen, only to realize later that it wasn't supposed to be part of your life's blueprint?
2. What were the consequences for you and for others of continuing to force it?
3. What did you learn from the experience?
4. What will you do differently going forward so that you can recognize your IKEA moments sooner and avoid needless suffering?

There's an old Yiddish proverb that goes, "If it's *bashert*, it's *bashert*." *Bashert* means "destiny." In other words, if it's meant to be, it's meant to be. How many times have you used that expression as a throwaway? We know we have a lot. But let's think more deeply about it. Imagine how your well-being would benefit if you really meant it. You'd take comfort in knowing that you had done your best, and you would accept the outcome regardless of what it was.

And, remember, just because you accept something doesn't mean you have to like it. In the words of Dale Carnegie, "Success is getting what you want. Happiness is wanting what you get."

STOPPING CAN BE A GREAT WAY TO START

In order to achieve certain goals, you may need to stop one activity before beginning another. Take credit card debt. There are three actions that apply to credit card debt: incurring, maintaining, and reducing. Incurring the debt is using your credit card but not paying it off at the end of the month. Maintaining the debt is paying the monthly finance charges but not reducing the principal balance or incurring any additional debt. Reducing is paying not only the finance charge but also the outstanding principal.

This is true with weight as well: incurring additional weight, maintaining a consistent weight, and reducing weight through diet and exercise. For those of you who have experienced chronic issues, whether it's living beyond your means, gaining weight, or whatever else, you may be better off first taking the little A. action of not exacerbating the situation. Give yourself the acknowledgement you deserve for not making it worse. With that under your belt, you can then take corrective action.

COMMITMENT AND ACCOUNTABILITY

Acting, as we have said, is the culmination of all the practices. For example, now that it's time to Act, you'll want to refer to Plan. If you've taken our planning suggestions, you've decided on the actions that you will take, along with the dates by which you will complete them. Whether they are big A. or little A. actions, you are moving forward in your life's journey as you minimize needless suffering and maximize well-being.

It is also effective to apply the practice of Reach Out to Act. Perhaps you want to take action but aren't sure how to follow through? Simple. Make a verbal or written commitment to someone who will hold you accountable. Don't give yourself a place to hide!

Recent research found that people who wrote down their goals, shared them with a friend, and sent weekly updates to that friend were on average 33 percent more successful in accomplishing their goals than those who merely formulated goals.[54]

Be sure to pick a supportive, yet firm, accountability buddy. Someone who will encourage you if you stumble but still hold you to your commitment. One of the best things about having people keep you on track is that you can celebrate with them when you finish!

Health and fitness initiatives are especially ideal for having a partner, whether it's a workout partner, someone to go to Weight Watchers with, or someone to quit smoking with. In addition to having reciprocal accountability, you have a built-in Reach Out person to encourage you. You are less likely to blow off going to the gym when you know your buddy is there waiting for you.

COMING FULL CIRCLE

Congratulations! You've now been exposed to the entire *What Matters?!* framework. It is our sincere hope that you will commit to incorporating the practices and mindsets into your everyday living. We once again invite you to take the quiz from Chapter 2, which will help you identify the areas you can strengthen in order to live what matters to you. After the quiz we've provided some reflection questions to help you solidify your learning and identify commitments for moving forward.

STOP AND ASK

I regularly stop and ask myself what is truly important.	Strongly Agree ☐	Agree ☐	Neutral ☐	Disagree ☐	Strongly Disagree ☐
I have a sense of purpose that guides what I do day-to-day.	Strongly Agree ☐	Agree ☐	Neutral ☐	Disagree ☐	Strongly Disagree ☐
Taking time for personal reflection is not optional; it is necessary for my well-being.	Strongly Agree ☐	Agree ☐	Neutral ☐	Disagree ☐	Strongly Disagree ☐

REACH IN

I feel grounded in who I am and how I take care of myself.	Strongly Agree ☐	Agree ☐	Neutral ☐	Disagree ☐	Strongly Disagree ☐
My negative self-talk rarely gets the better of me.	Strongly Agree ☐	Agree ☐	Neutral ☐	Disagree ☐	Strongly Disagree ☐
I know what I need to do to recharge my batteries when I'm feeling depleted.	Strongly Agree ☐	Agree ☐	Neutral ☐	Disagree ☐	Strongly Disagree ☐

I accept, without frustration or resentment, that there are things in life that I cannot change.	Strongly Agree ☐	Agree ☐	Neutral ☐	Disagree ☐	Strongly Disagree ☐

REACH OUT

Although I have a group of family and friends, I often feel lonely.	Strongly Agree ☐	Agree ☐	Neutral ☐	Disagree ☐	Strongly Disagree ☐
It's easier to figure things out by myself rather than include others in the process.	Strongly Agree ☐	Agree ☐	Neutral ☐	Disagree ☐	Strongly Disagree ☐
When faced with challenges, I rarely turn to friends or family for ideas, advice, and encouragement.	Strongly Agree ☐	Agree ☐	Neutral ☐	Disagree ☐	Strongly Disagree ☐

I rarely call at least one friend or family member every day just to say hello.	Strongly Agree ☐	Agree ☐	Neutral ☐	Disagree ☐	Strongly Disagree ☐

PLAN

I want to make changes in my life but am unsure how to proceed.	Strongly Agree ☐	Agree ☐	Neutral ☐	Disagree ☐	Strongly Disagree ☐
I seldom prioritize how I spend my time.	Strongly Agree ☐	Agree ☐	Neutral ☐	Disagree ☐	Strongly Disagree ☐
I'm often so busy it feels like my life is running me instead of me running my life.	Strongly Agree ☐	Agree ☐	Neutral ☐	Disagree ☐	Strongly Disagree ☐
I struggle with deciding what I will say yes to and what I will say no to.	Strongly Agree ☐	Agree ☐	Neutral ☐	Disagree ☐	Strongly Disagree ☐

ACT

I like to wait until everything is perfectly aligned rather than start and risk failure.	Strongly Agree ☐	Agree ☐	Neutral ☐	Disagree ☐	Strongly Disagree ☐
I seldom follow through on what I say I am going to do.	Strongly Agree ☐	Agree ☐	Neutral ☐	Disagree ☐	Strongly Disagree ☐
Most of my choices are based on what I fear rather than creating what I want	Strongly Agree ☐	Agree ☐	Neutral ☐	Disagree ☐	Strongly Disagree ☐
If I died tomorrow, I'd regret not having done what I really wanted to do.	Strongly Agree ☐	Agree ☐	Neutral ☐	Disagree ☐	Strongly Disagree ☐

MINDSETS

CURIOSITY: I view the world with wonder and open- mindedness.	Strongly Agree	Agree	Neutral	Disagree	Strongly Disagree
	☐	☐	☐	☐	☐

SELF-HONESTY: I tell myself the truth without judgment or negativity.	Strongly Agree	Agree	Neutral	Disagree	Strongly Disagree
	☐	☐	☐	☐	☐

HUMOR: I don't take myself or the world too seriously.	Strongly Agree	Agree	Neutral	Disagree	Strongly Disagree
	☐	☐	☐	☐	☐

GRATITUDE: I appreciate what and who I have in my life.	Strongly Agree	Agree	Neutral	Disagree	Strongly Disagree
	☐	☐	☐	☐	☐

KINDNESS: I'm compassionate toward myself and others.	Strongly Agree	Agree	Neutral	Disagree	Strongly Disagree
	☐	☐	☐	☐	☐

WORKING IT

1. Which of the *What Matters?!* practices and mindsets are you most committed to bringing into your life?
2. How will strengthening these focus areas help improve your well-being?
3. What will you do to include these practices and mindsets in your daily routine? What specific actions will you take?
4. Who will you Reach Out to for support?

RICH'S STORY: GOING ALL IN

We chose to feature Rich here because, even though What Matters?! *is about decreasing stress and increasing well-being, we all have our own definition of well-being—some people thrive on pushing themselves. Remember,* What Matters?! *is personal.*

If Rich had a mantra, it would probably be "go big or go home." He has been happily married for more than twenty years and is the proud parent of twins, a boy and a girl. Rich has been very successful in his career, having worked in consulting as well as management positions for multinational companies. He has also traveled extensively, both domestically and internationally.

Rich likes to be challenged in his work, and he thrives outside of his comfort zone. In early 2004, a friend courted him to join a venture that he was starting with some other colleagues. They were planning on developing large-scale residential properties and wanted to start a subsidiary business unit to manage the properties. Rich would be the chief operating officer. After turning down the offer several times, he Reached In and decided he had nothing to lose by trying it out. He Acted and took the job for a trial period of one year.

A year turned into two, and eventually after six years, he took over as president of the division, where he made the property management firm even more successful. However, he found himself becoming restless. By this time, the twins were in college. Rich and his wife had planned for the expense of their children's education, and given his success, many people in his place would have started slowing down.

Rich Stopped and Asked himself why he was feeling unhappy with his work. It was then that he realized he was feeling boxed in. His vision as president for the property management firm was broader than that of its current owner. With his hands tied, he decided to give his notice, but at the last minute, he Reached In and reconsidered. Having been a part of the organization from its inception, he cared deeply about the people he worked with. If he left the company, the owners might sell off the division to a larger property management company. This would put the employees in jeopardy.

Through self-honesty, Rich realized he didn't want to leave the business that he had helped build. In fact, what he really wanted was to buy the division and turn it into his own company. Which is exactly what he did. Immediately after buying the division, he renamed and rebranded it. His company today continues to grow steadily, serving condominium, apartment, and commercial properties. It invests heavily in technology and green initiatives to run the most efficient and environmentally friendly buildings in the Southeast.

Rich exemplifies how decisive action allows you to live What Matters?! And he shows that, for some people, well-being is achieved by taking on more responsibility, not less.

CONCLUSION

We begin this final chapter with one of our favorite quotations, courtesy of twentieth-century author Christopher Morley. For us, it sums up the spirit of *What Matters?!*

There is only one success—to be able to spend your life in your own way.

Our sincere hope is that the *What Matters?!* framework will provide you with the tools to find the manner of living that works for you. The goal of the *What Matters?!* approach is to lead you to a fully engaged life. Choice is the key to your well-being. By mindfully choosing and then taking action, you will live your best life.

Remember, you can Stop and Ask *What Matters?!* in any situation. You can Reach In and align your body, mind, and spirit with what is right for you, then you can Reach Out for help. You can draw up a Plan and put that plan into Action with some accountability. All the while, you can incorporate the mindsets of Humor,

Self-honesty, Gratitude, Kindness, and Curiosity to support you in each one of these practices. You also know now the obstacles you might face along the way and how to overcome them.

A BETTER WORLD

In the introduction we mentioned that asking what matters not only helps you thrive, but it may even improve our world. Being at your best, you inspire others to achieve the same well-being in their own lives, because it is infectious. Imagine living in a world of fully engaged people. If you ask us, that's certainly a whole lot more satisfying than being surrounded by stressed-out people who are just trying to get by.

Along with inspiring others through your well-being, our hope is that you actively Reach Out and share the *What Matters?!* framework with the people in your life. You don't have to be a *What Matters?!* evangelist (although we would LOVE that), but this is a community learning model and our hope is that it will become second nature to not only live consciously yourself, but to help others do so as well. Our website, www.askwhat matters.com, has an overview of the *What Matters?!* approach along with a number of tools to help implement the practices and mindsets.

WHAT MATTERS?! CONVERSATIONS

A very simple way of helping others find their path to well-being is through *What Matters?!* conversations. We stumbled onto this practice one fall afternoon in Joe Coffee Shop in Provincetown, Massachusetts. After ordering his favorite muffin and coffee, Paul turned to the server and said, "Do you mind if I ask you something that you may find a bit odd?" Being Provincetown, a place known for its unconventionality, the woman responded, "Honey, you can't possibly ask me anything odder than I've already heard! Go for it." With that, Paul asked her, "What matters to you?" At first she stared blankly. "What do you mean?" Paul responded, "What matters to you in life?"

What ensued was a five-minute conversation (the shop was pretty empty) during which the woman shared all about the things most important to her. At the end of the dialogue, she declared, "That was really cool." Without any prompting, the server then approached her coworker and asked, "What matters?" It was contagious.

Since then we've made it a regular practice to engage people in *What Matters?!* conversations. In fact, we begin all of our workshops with participants asking one another, "What matters?" The very simple act of discussing the question without judging the responses fosters engagement, interpersonal connection, and well-being.

So, if you do nothing else after having read this book, we invite you to simply Stop and Ask yourself and others what matters on a regular basis.

Here's a tool to help you engage in a basic *What Matters?!* conversation. Why not try it at the dinner table? How about with your team at work?

WHAT MATTERS?! DISCUSSION ACTIVITY

OBJECTIVE

The purpose of this activity is to:

- help each member of a group (e.g., family, work team) to gain clarity about what matters to them
- foster an understanding within the group about what matters to each member
- identify things that group members can do or say to encourage and support each individual in living what matters to them

PRIOR TO THE DISCUSSION

- Select someone who will facilitate the activity. It doesn't necessarily have to be the person with the most authority (e.g., parent or team leader).

- Inform group members that there will be an upcoming discussion which will give them a chance to get better acquainted. Tell them that each member of the group will be given the floor to share the things that are most important to them—"what matters."

- In preparation for the conversation, invite people to reflect on *What Matters?!* to them in the various aspects of their lives.

AT THE MEETING

1. Request that everyone be curious and as open as possible (i.e., suspend judgment). Let them know that there is no right or wrong in what anyone has to say.

2. Explain that each person will have the floor for up to five minutes. During that time, he or she will share what matters, then the group can ask clarifying questions.

3. Ask for a volunteer who is willing to go first.

4. After the individual shares, allow members of the group to ask that person questions. *DO NOT ALLOW COMMENTS. THIS IS ABOUT QUESTIONS ONLY.*

5. Ask if anyone would like to share comments/reactions about what they learned about the group member who has just shared. Set the ground rule that the comments cannot be judgmental.

6. Ask the person whose turn it is if he or she has any other final comments or questions.

7. Repeat this process with each member

8. Once all members of the group have had a chance to share, open the floor to discuss what it was like to both share what matters to them and listen to what matters to others.

Andrea and Steven's Story: Intentional Living

When Texas native Andrea met Steven from Scotland, their connection was immediate and strong. They quickly realized that with some intentional planning and mindful choosing, they could build an extraordinary life together.

Although they came from different parts of the world, Andrea and Steven had very similar backgrounds. They both grew up in strong, healthy families where their parents served as great role models on how to be a supportive parent and life partner. Andrea and Steven also had a deep connection to their Jewish faith and their community—two things they believed helped the world be a better place for all families. They had many heart-to-heart conversations about what they wanted for themselves as a couple, including their vision of the future and the values they would instill in their children if they were so blessed.

After marrying, they relocated to London where they both found jobs. They loved the excitement of the bustling city and everything it had to offer. They also travelled extensively throughout Europe. They talked about mindfully choosing a life that was aligned with their goals and values. Although they loved London and all that came with it, they also knew that they would want to slow down when they started a family. As glamorous and cosmopolitan as it was, London also had its downsides. Observing young families in the city, Andrea and Steven realized that simple trips to the grocery store were complicated and stressful. They also watched colleagues tutoring their five-year-olds in order to get them into the right schools. And although they were doing well financially, their affluence did not reflect their own happy childhoods nor did it fit the intentional life they wanted. They weren't judging other people's choices, but Andrea and Steven wanted to choose their own path for their family. They were blessed with three girls in four years.

A visit to Andrea's cousin in Jacksonville, Florida, ended up being a fortuitous trip. Andrea's cousin had always been a mentor to her, and during her visit, Andrea realized that life in Jacksonville had many of the attributes that Steven and Andrea were looking for. There was a wholesomeness to the area. There was a warm Jewish community set in a warm larger community in general. The city had a slower pace than London, and it wasn't overly planned. They also liked the warmer climate—flip flops bring out the best in people!

They bought a nice home in which to raise their family. They intentionally chose a home where their three girls could share a bedroom, as both Andrea and Steven had done growing up with their siblings. They continue to carefully choose everything from chores to cell phones so that their children don't feel entitled and remain grounded.

Annette Funicello said, "Life doesn't have to be perfect to be wonderful." Andrea admits that her life is hardly perfect, yet she is still happy, because she had deep, meaningful conversations with Steven before getting married, and she continues to be present and mindful in her daily choices. Andrea says, "I wish people would remember to plan for their marriage as well as their wedding."

BRINGING WHAT MATTERS?! INTO YOUR LIFE: AT HOME

Imagine having regular *What Matters?!* conversations at your dinner table. Your family would have a common language for raising issues—everything from family vacations to end-of-life decisions. And with regular dialogue, you would all have the tools to help each other when one of you stumbles on your *What Matters?!* journey.

Imagine being able to have a *What Matters?!* conversation when your teenage son comes home from school and locks himself in his room. You know something is wrong, but you are lucky if he talks to you when he's in a good mood, let alone when he's upset. What would it be like if your family had a plan for situations like this? How much would your stress decrease if you could slip a picture of an octopus eating pizza under his door with a note saying "YOU Matter!"—a predetermined ice breaker to convey, "Let's get some pizza and talk about what's going on." How would it feel to be able to turn your child's pain into a supportive, problem-solving opportunity? Maybe you could help him focus on the good in his life. Maybe you could reframe his current struggle in the context of life beyond the tumultuous teenage years. Maybe he would realize that, although you don't know what it's like to be a teenager today, you were still once his age and now have the benefit of hindsight and experience.

AT WORK

Managers, picture using *What Matters?!* at work. Think about enriching your career development conversations by openly discussing with your employees how their career aspirations integrate with the bigger scheme of their lives. Imagine using the *What Matters?!* framework to help coach your employees through stressful situations.

Envision the cohesion, and yes, even intimacy, that would result from colleagues asking and hearing what matters to one another. And at the collective level, imagine leading a group dialogue where you coalesce around what matters to your department, work group, or team as a whole. Think about the level of alignment and common culture you could create in your organization by introducing the *What Matters?!* framework—a shorthand language for creativity, problem-solving, and conflict management. A shared mindset of open and honest communication with no blame or judgment.

Imagine walking into work and your team is precipitously close to missing a major deadline. What would a *What Matters?!* conversation look like in this situation? Maybe people would talk about what is going right in the project. Maybe you would figure out some steps to bypass or resources to bring in to ensure you meet the deadline. Maybe you would decide to approach the higher ups and explain that although you may miss the deadline, the end result will be worth it—something that everyone can rally behind.

ROGER'S STORY: CHOOSING THE RIGHT EMPLOYER

Roger was a successful attorney on track to becoming partner at a prestigious law firm. He was the father of three small boys, but he and his wife, Louise, had decided that his long work hours would be worth it in the long run. They had a nice home in a town with great public schools, and Louise was able to stay at home with the boys full-time. Then one day, Roger realized that he was missing special moments in his sons' lives that could never be recaptured. In particular, Roger wanted the chance to coach their baseball teams. He went to one of the senior partners at his firm and expressed his concern.

The senior partner, however, firmly believed that Roger should stick with the demanding hours—that it would be worth it in the end. Once Roger made partner, he said, his income would allow him to easily meet the financial obligation of the boys' college education as well as enjoy expensive family vacations and a comfortable retirement. The senior partner also told him that becoming partner meant trading the long billable hours for work dinners and weekend golf outings with clients. In other words, Roger's responsibilities would change but not his time commitment.

Roger and Louise saw this as a Stop and Ask moment. What mattered to them the most at this point? They agreed that the answer was Roger spending quality time with his boys—something he could never get back.

Roger and Louise sat down and decided it was time for a change. Roger's plan ever since he was an undergrad was to make partner in a law firm. He Reached In to figure out what he wanted to do now. He still loved legal work, so he knew he didn't want to make a drastic change. He and his family had also grown accustomed to a certain standard of living and he didn't want to give that up, either. Roger wasn't afraid of hard work and actually thrived on a certain amount of pressure. What he didn't want was to be responsible for tracking a certain number of billable hours. He decided his plan was to find an in-house counsel position where he wouldn't have to worry about logging billable hours. There were plenty of large corporations in his geographical area and many of the companies offered stock and bonus plans that were as enticing as the benefits he would have received as partner in the firm. Roger Reached Out and engaged his network—former colleagues, friends from college and law school, as well as a few professors whom he had strong ties with.

Soon, Roger found an in-house counsel job with a prominent financial services company in the same city where he and his family lived. His job package included a great salary, stock, and bonus structure to compensate for the demands and pressure that came with such a high-profile position. Roger was careful to thoroughly address the time commitment the firm expected from him. As in-house counsel he would oversee all SEC filings; it appeared that other than the three weeks leading up to the quarterly filing periods, he would not be asked to sacrifice time from his family.

During the interview process, he was told that the company expected him to work hard, but unlike a firm with billable hours, the emphasis was on performance and effectiveness. If employees had family commitments, then by all means they should take care of them. That being said, the company trusted that its employees would get their work done.

As Roger sat in his final interview with the president of the firm, he was asked if he had any questions. He spoke candidly: he was looking for a long-term work environment that would appreciate his commitment to his family and his personal wishes. He said, "What matters most to me at this point is spending time with my boys. Will I be able to coach my sons' baseball teams?"

The boss's response came as a pleasant surprise. "Roger, we want you to work here for a very long time. We want you to make this your career. And if coaching Little League is important to you, then it is important to our company, too."

GOING DEEPER WITH WHAT MATTERS?! CONVERSATIONS

Beyond simply asking "What matters?" in a general discussion, you can also use the *What Matters?!* framework to engage others on a specific topic. Is there a mutual decision that needs to be made? A conflict needing resolution? Whether at home, at work, or in your community, using the *What Matters?!* framework can protect the well-being of both parties in the dialogue itself as well as in the outcome generated. Here's a tool to assist:

WHAT MATTERS?! CONVERSATION GUIDE

PURPOSE

Use this tool to guide a conversation regarding a topic where there are varying viewpoints.

1. Let's start by agreeing to be curious and kind to one another in this discussion. Let's also agree to be as honest with ourselves as we can while finding humor where appropriate.

2. **STOP AND ASK:** What matters to each of us individually in this specific situation? What matters to us collectively?

3. **REACH IN:** How do we each need to adapt our thoughts and feelings to ensure we are mutually aligned in this situation?

4. **REACH OUT:** Who else do we need to bring into this conversation?

5. **PLAN:** What are the specific steps we need to take? Who will do them and by when?

6. **ACT:** How will we know that we have put our plan into action? What can we do to hold ourselves accountable?

7. What are we grateful for in this situation and how we conducted this discussion?

IN YOUR COMMUNITY

In addition to bringing the *What Matters?!* approach to your own life, to your family, and at work, we urge you to bring it into your greater community. As we have said throughout this book, *What Matters?!* is a shared learning model. We can all learn from and teach each other. The Reach Out practice reminds us to routinely ask for and offer help. Beyond this, we believe that we need to work together to improve the status quo. Although we may have our differences, we know that ultimately what unites us as people is greater than what divides us.

When we join forces for the common good, the possibilities are endless. Imagine each of us uniting our unique skillsets with the complimentary skills of others, whether it's putting on a bake sale or building a new ball field. In the end, you have not only improved your community, but you feel proud of what you have accomplished together.

RANDI AND BOB'S STORY: BRINGING A COMMUNITY TOGETHER

Randi and Bob moved to Boston's South End in 1986 with their seven-year-old son, Keith. They had been living in the suburbs but were drawn to the South End because of its rich cultural history and vibrant community characterized by diversity of race, income, and gender/sexual identity.

On the day they moved into their home, the president of the Blackstone Franklin Square Neighborhood Association (BFSNA) swung by to welcome them and encourage them to join the organization. At the time, there were twenty-two different neighborhood associations, each representing a specific area of the South End. Randi and Bob immediately joined the BFSNA, with Bob serving as president for two years and then Randi for eight years.

The area was facing major challenges. The Washington Street corridor was blighted after the termination and removal of the elevated Orange Line MBTA subway service. Also, the area had only a 7 percent owner-occupancy rate, many empty buildings, seven acres of parcels that needed to be developed, and was known primarily for drugs and prostitution. Every morning Randi was faced with a Stop and Ask moment about how she could improve her neighborhood. She would wake up early, put on rubber gloves, and go to the bus stop to pick up syringe needles and condoms prior to bringing Keith.

Randi was happy with the progress BFSNA was making. However, she felt that the only way to truly revitalize the Washington Street area would be to join forces with the other neighborhood associations. Randi Reached Out to the presidents of five other neighborhood associations that abutted Washington Street and asked them to join her in a meeting with Thomas Menino, the new mayor of Boston.

In that meeting with Mayor Menino, Randi and the others shared their experiences and hopes for the neighborhood. Mayor Menino was interested in their ideas and said he would do everything in his power to support them.

The six neighborhood groups came together and worked as one. For the first time, neighborhood associations, not-for-profits, and businesses worked together to reclaim Washington Street and restore its grandeur. Their monthly meetings moved throughout the various neighborhoods so that all members were familiar with each other's areas and could work as one with a larger vision.

Together, they started with little A. actions, like removing barbed wire, painting mailboxes, and cleaning up graffiti. These small actions created a sense of pride in the neighborhood. To help with this effort Mayor Menino appointed the Washington Street Task Force, and made Randi the chair. The group started working with the city and the Boston Redevelopment Authority to change zoning and entice redevelopment of vacant lots and buildings. The new zoning increased the height of buildings on Washington Street, with retail on the ground floor and housing above to create a vibrant neighborhood and active streetscape.

Their big P. plans included directing the use of the $52 million in federal funds that had been set aside for infrastructure improvements along Washington Street as part of the relocation of the Orange Line. Their plans led to action, as buildings were renovated and empty parcels developed and the streets adorned with brick sidewalks, acorn lights, and elm trees. The group was then renamed the Washington Gateway Main Street, which won many national awards and became a model for the inclusionary process in urban development. Randi shares, "The transformation of Washington Street was beyond our imagination. We credit the success with staying focused on the task at hand, tapping into our strengths as a community, and reaching out for help when needed."

BIG "I" INVITATION AND ONE FINAL QUESTION

Before we say goodbye (for now), we have one final question for you. It's a biggie, so get ready: "What are we here for anyway?" (And you thought *What Matters?!* was tough!)

Our premise for writing *What Matters?!* is that we humans are on this earth to be generative. It's about the legacy we leave. Whether that legacy is creating art, developing technology, making music, constructing buildings, planting gardens, or nurturing relationships, we, as a race, are more likely to be generative when we individually and collectively are in a state of well-being as opposed to one of stress and angst. Well-being gives us access to our unique strengths so that we can make our best contribution to civilization. Plus, when I'm at my best, I create an environment that allows you to be at your best, and vice versa.

The world is complicated. We know that we cannot completely escape stress and angst. That being "reality," we hope we have offered you a human technology that helps you to experience life not as a struggle to overcome but as a positive personal journey for you and everyone else.

ENDNOTES

1. Jeff Davidson, *The Complete Idiot's Guide to Getting Things Done* (New York: Alpha Books, 2005).
2. "What to Do When There Are Too Many Product Choices on the Store Shelves?" *Consumer Reports*, January 2014, http://www.consumerreports.org/cro/magazine/2014/03/too-many-product-choices-in-supermarkets/index.htm.
3. *Business Insider*, May 16, 2012.
4. Lisa O'Kelly, "Interview with Daniel J. Levitin," *The Guardian*, January 18, 2015.
5. Statistic Brain Research Institute, American Institute of Stress, New York, October 19, 2015.
6. Brigid Schulte, *Overwhelmed: Work, Love, and Play When No One Has the Time* (New York: Sarah Crichton Books, 2014).
7. Ibid.
8. American Institute of Stress, http://www.stress.org/workplace-stress/.
9. Daniel Goleman, "What Makes a Leader?" *Harvard Business Review*, January 2004.
10. Brigid Schulte, *Overwhelmed: Work, Love, and Play When No One Has the Time* (New York: Sarah Crichton Books, 2014).
11. http://www.christiancinema.com/catalog/newsdesk_info.php?newsdesk_id=3216
12. Dustin Wood, Peter Harms, Simine Vazire, "Perceiver Effects as Projective Tests: What Your Perceptions of Others Say About You." *Digital Commons@ University of Nebraska-Lincoln*, January 2010.
13. http://thisibelieve.org/essay/15753/.

14. Russ Harris, *The Happiness Trap: How to Stop Struggling and Start Living: A Guide to Act* (Boston: Trumpeter Books, An Imprint of Shambala Publications, Inc. 2008).

15. Jay Earley and Bonnie J. Weiss, *Freedom from Your Inner Critic: A Self-therapy Approach* (Boulder: Sounds True, Inc., 2013).

16. Richard Carson, *Taming Your Gremlin: A Surprisingly Simple Method for Getting Out of Your Own Way* (New York: HarperCollins, 2003).

17. Henry Kimsey-House, Karen Kimsey-House, Phillip Sandahl, and Laura Whitworth, *Co-Active Coaching: Changing Business, Transforming Lives* (Boston: Nicholas Brealey Publishing, 2011).

18. Center for Right Relationship, http://www.crrglobal.com.

19. Cynthia Loy-Darst, http://www.theinspirationpoint.com.

20. Source: Dr. John Kenworthy, http://gapps5.com/10-cognitive-distortions

21. "Neuroscientists Discover Brain Area Responsible for Fear of Losing Money," Phys.org, February 8, 2010, http://phys.org/news/2010-02-neuroscientists-brain-area-responsible-money.html.

22. Lydia Saad, "Americans' Money Worries Unchanged from 2014," *Gallup*, April 20, 2015, http://www.gallup.com/poll/182768/americans-money-worries-unchanged-2014.aspx.

23. http://www.goodreads.com/quotes/523350-if-you-are-depressed-you-are-living-in-the-past.

24. Pema Chödrön, *The Pocket Pema Chodron*, ed. Eden Steinberg (Boston: Shambhala, 2010).

25. Scott Plous, *The Psychology of Judgment and Decision Making* (New York: McGraw-Hill, 1993).

26. http://www.goodreads.com/quotes/485998-what-you-resist-persists.

27. Byron Katie, *Loving What Is: Four Questions That Can Change Your Life* (New York: Three Rivers Press, 2002).

28. Richard Carson, *Taming Your Gremlin: A Surprisingly Simple Method for Getting Out of Your Own Way* (New York: HarperCollins, 2003).

29. Julia Cameron, *The Artist's Way: A Spiritual Path to Higher Creativity* (New York: Jeremy P. Tarcher/Putnam, 1992).

30. Russ Harris, *The Happiness Trap: How to Stop Struggling and Start Living: A Guide to Act* (Boston: Trumpeter Books, An Imprint of Shambala Publications, Inc. 2008).

31. Stan Slap, *Bury My Heart in Conference Room B: The Unbeatable Impact of Truly Committed Managers* (New York: Penguin Group, 2010).

32. Kelly Wilson and Troy DuFrene, *The Wisdom to Know the Difference: An Acceptance and Commitment Workbook for Overcoming Substance Abuse* (Oakland: New Harbinger Publications, 2012).

33. Ruth Beckman Murray, Judith Proctor Zentner, and Richard Yakimo, *Health Promotions Strategies through the Life Span* (New Jersey: Prentice Hall, 2008).

34. "Laughter is the Best Medicine for Your Heart," July 14, 2009 Press Release, University of Maryland Medical Center.

35. Yagana Shah, "New Study Proves That Laughter Really Is the Best Medicine," *Huffington Post,* April 22, 2014. http://www.huffingtonpost.com/2014/04/22/laughter-and-memory_n_5192086.html.

36. David R. Hamilton, *Why Kindness Is Good for You* (California: Hay House, 2010).

37. Allan Luks and Peggy Payne, *The Healing Power of Doing Good* (Nebraska: iUniverse, 1991).

38. Pema Chödrön, *Comfortable with Uncertainty* (Boston: Shambhala Publications, 2002).

39. Todd Kashdan, "The Power of Curiosity," *Experience Life,* May 2010.

40. Christopher Peterson and Martin Seligman, *Character Strengths and Virtues: A Handbook and Classification* (New York: American Psychological Association/Oxford University Press, 2004).

41. Todd Kashdan, "The Power of Curiosity," *Experience Life,* May 2010.

42. Robert A. Emmons, *Thanks! How Practicing Gratitude Can Make You Happier* (New York: Houghton Mifflin, 2008).

43. Greater Good Science Center at the University of California, Berkeley.

44. Wayne Baker, *United America* (Canton, MI: Read the Spirit Books, 2014).

45. Greater Good Science Center at the University of California, Berkeley.

46. Adam Grant, "Givers Take All: The Hidden Dimension of Corporate Culture," *McKinsey Quarterly,* April 2014.

47. http://www.meetup.com.

48. http://www.goodreads.com/quotes/93999-when-a-great-moment-knocks-on-the-door-of-your.

49. Eckhart Tolle, *Stillness Speaks* (Novato, CA: New World Library, 2003).

50. Charles Wheelan, *10 ½ Things No Commencement Speaker Has Ever Said* (New York: W.W. Norton & Company, 2012).

51. http://www.goodreads.com/author/quotes/334180.Tony_Blair.

52. Hara Estroff Marano, "Procrastination: Ten Things to Know," *Psychology Today,* August 23, 2003.

53. Oxford Dictionaries, http://www.oxforddictionaries.com

54. Nancy Anderson, "Five Ways to Make Your New Year's Resolutions Stick," *Forbes,* January 3, 2013, http://www.forbes.com/sites/financialfinesse/2013/01/03/5-ways-to-make-your-new-years-resolutions-stick/#740132606c57.

ACKNOWLEDGMENTS

To properly thank all those who helped with this book, we would have to thank every person we have ever met, since this book is an amalgamation of everything we have learned. Short of that, we would like to thank our family and friends for their boundless love and support.

Thank you, Janelle Hoyland, for giving us the mandate to create a path for traversing these times and for encouraging us to own this work.

To our early advisors: James Chung, Jean DiGiovanna, Charlie Jacobs, Barb Levison, Lee Levison, Christine Petersen, Theresa Moulton, Beth Shapiro, Risa Sherman, Andrea Shlipak-Mail, and Julie Silver for helping us create the *What Matters?!* approach.

To our beta readers: the "fabulous" Debra Gold, "beta" Barb Levison, Bonnie Maitlen, Martin McGovern, Christine Petersen, and Susan Robinson for your insightful and heartfelt feedback.

Thank you Dorothy Skelley for your insights and commitment.

To those who so openly and willingly shared personal stories so we could illustrate the benefits of the What Matters?! approach, we are so very grateful.

Thanks to Carol Lundeen for the wonderful photo of us and Brando—you made us look good!

Thank you to our amazing graphics team: Jennifer Smith-Little, for creating such an awesome book cover and for developing our overall visual identity; Steven Mousterakis, for generously donating your time and mastery to create the original What Matters?! visual; Dave Lennon, for jumpstarting our initial creative process; and Molly Regan, for the finishing touches.

Thank you, Lisa Mauro, for your counsel and inspiration.

Robert Haas and Geoffry McEnany, you are true gifts to the mental health profession. Thank you for helping us get through the dark times and for being here to celebrate the good.

Frances, thanks for inspiring us, making us laugh, and being the glue.

Thank you, Mary Beaulieu, Lisa Kelly-Croswell, Rabbi Neal Gold, Stephanie Khurana, Phil Sandahl, and Dr. Nick van Dam, for your generous endorsements.

To Stuart Horwitz of Book Architecture, our awesome collaborator: we are thrilled with the outcome and had a great time working with you. THANK YOU FOR HELPING US PULL IT ALL TOGETHER!

C. S. Plocher, thank you for your masterful editing. There's no one better!

Thank you Ronda Rawlins and the team at 1106 Design for creating a layout that expresses the tone of our work.

To Paul's coaches through the years: Matthew Rochte, Ron Renaud, and Alan Seale. Laura Whitworth, your fierceness and commitment to humankind has left an indelible imprint. You are dearly missed. And, Ken Mossman, for helping to navigate the biggest breakthroughs of all.

Another shout-out to Christine Petersen for always going the extra mile.

Once again to Barb Levison for your never-ending encouragement, candor, and dedication. "It's a thing!"

And finally to our great and dear friend, the amazing and talented Beth Shapiro, for all your wisdom, great writing, and endless love and support. We are blessed to have you in our lives.

To all you mentioned and to those we may have missed, we thank you wholeheartedly for joining us on this amazing journey.

WITH GRATITUDE AND LOVE,
—DAVID AND PAUL

WORKSHOPS & COACHING SERVICES WITH DAVID AND PAUL

Looking to do more with *What Matters?!* We are thrilled to offer the following services for corporate and workgroups, community and faith-based organizations, not-for-profits, academic institutions, or any other group that would be interested:

- Two Hour *What Matters?!* Jump-Start Workshop
- One and Two Day *What Matters?!* Intensive Workshops
- Customized Workshops for Organizations
- Speaking Engagements
- Individual Coaching
- Team and Workgroup Coaching

For further information please email us at info@askwhatmatters.com or call 508-413-9280.

We look forward to the opportunity to work with you!

—DAVID AND PAUL

ABOUT THE AUTHORS

Co-authors Paul Sherman and David Garten are a married couple who coach individuals and organizations (corporate, community, and faith-based) around the world. Their passion and mission is to help people live their best lives by eliminating needless suffering. They believe that we all do better when we work together and that we can all learn from and teach each other.

Paul Sherman is a certified professional coach and workshop leader specializing in individual, team, and organizational performance. Over his twenty-five-year career he has brought his unique blend of people and business acumen to over fifty major corporations and government agencies worldwide. Described by *Forbes* as a "miracle medium," Paul is a pioneer in the emerging field of Team Coaching and is a featured speaker and writer on the topic.

In addition to his extensive coaching and consulting, Paul has held key management positions at Cambridge Technology Partners, Blue Cross Blue Shield of Massachusetts, Amherst Consulting Group, and Vertex Pharmaceuticals. A summa cum laude, Phi Beta Kappa graduate of Harvard University, Paul holds a bachelor of arts in psychology and a master's in human resources education from Boston University.

David Garten started his career in commercial lending and private banking. He has also worked in marketing and sales in software and high-tech. A serial entrepreneur, David has been involved in the start-up and growth of companies in the gift, personal care, and service industries. With his long-standing interest in social justice and strong communities, he was Director of Housing Development for a nonprofit that developed more than five hundred units of mixed-income housing in the Boston area. David holds a bachelor of science in business administration from Babson College and is a certified team coach.

Paul and David are grateful to live in Provincetown, Massachusetts, with their rescue dog, Brando.

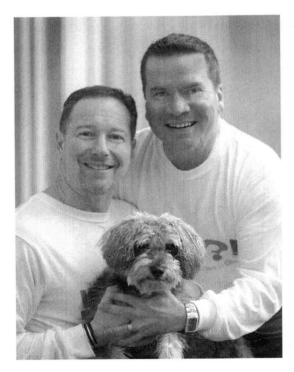